The American Cancer Society
LYMPHEDEMA

Results from a Workshop on Breast Cancer
Treatment-Related Lymphedema
and
Lymphedema Resource Guide

Originally published in
Cancer: Interdisciplinary International Journal
of the American Cancer Society,
Volume 83, 1998, pages 2775-2890.

The American Cancer Society
Lymphedema
Results from a Workshop on Breast Cancer
Treatment-Related Lymphedema
and Lymphedema Resource Guide

Jeanne Petrek, MD
Peter I. Pressman, MD
Robert A. Smith, PhD

This material was originally published in Cancer: The Interdisciplinary International Journal of the American Cancer Society. The journal is the only appropriate literature citation for the articles printed in this book.

Cancer 1998; 83: 2775-2890.

The American Cancer Society
LYMPHEDEMA

Results from a Workshop on Breast Cancer
Treatment-Related Lymphedema
and
Lymphedema Resource Guide

Jeanne Petrek, MD
Director, Surgical Program of the Lauder Breast
Center, Memorial Sloan Kettering Cancer Center

Peter I. Pressman, MD
Clinical Professor of Surgery, Albert Einstein School
of Medicine, Attending Surgeon, Beth Israel Medical
Center and Lenox Hill Hospital

Robert A. Smith, PhD
Director, Cancer Screening,
American Cancer Society

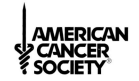

AMERICAN
CANCER
SOCIETY®

Hope. Progress. Answers.

#42646848

-06

iv

Interdisciplinary International Journal of the American Cancer Society

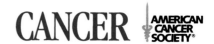

Contents 83/12 Supplement
December 15, 1998

Contents 83/12 Supplement December 15, 1998

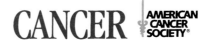

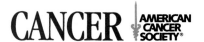

Contents 83/12 Supplement December 15, 1998

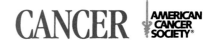

Interdisciplinary International Journal of the American Cancer Society

Workgroup Reports

Interdisciplinary International Journal of the American Cancer Society

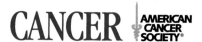

Contents 83/12 Supplement December 15, 1998

CANCER (ISSN 0008-543X) is published semi-monthly except tri-monthly in February, April, June, August, October, and December, for the American Cancer Society by Wiley-Liss, Inc., a subsidiary of John Wiley & Sons, Inc., 605 Third Avenue, New York, NY 10158-0012, (212) 850-6995, toll-free (800) 511-3989. Periodicals postage paid at New York, NY, and at additional mailing offices. Send subscription inquiries to: John Wiley & Sons, Inc., Subscription Department, 605 Third Avenue, 9th Floor, New York, NY 10158-0012. Annual subscription prices: 30 issues (includes 6 issues of CANCER CYTOPATHOLOGY section): Institutional rate: Within United States, $367.00; Canada and Mexico, $507.00; all other countries except Japan, $585.00. Individual rate: Within United States, $202.00; Canada and Mexico, $287.00; all other countries except Japan, $397.00. 24 issues—CANCER only—Individual rate: Within United States, $150.00; Canada and Mexico, $235.00; all other countries except Japan, $297.00. 6 issues—CANCER CYTOPATHOLOGY only—Individual rate: Within United States, $65.00; Canada and Mexico, $65.00; all other countries except Japan, $100.00. Add 7% GST for all Canadian orders; Wiley's GST number is R891028052. All subscriptions outside the U.S. will be sent by air. Payment must be made in U.S. dollars drawn on a U.S. bank. All payments for CANCER must be sent to John Wiley & Sons, Inc., P.O. Box 7247-7126, Philadelphia, PA 19170-7126.

ADVERTISING Advertising inquiries should be directed to: Noel White and Associates, 307 East 90th Street, Suite 7e, New York, NY 10128, (212) 876-6199, fax (212) 876-8120. Advertisements appearing in CANCER and the statements, representations and views expressed therein are the statements, representations and views of the individual advertisers only. The American Cancer Society, the Editors, the members of the Editorial Boards, and the Publisher make no warranty as to the accuracy of any information set forth therein, and accept no responsibility or liability for any inaccuracy or errors and omissions, or for any damage or injury to persons or property arising out of any such advertisements.

CHANGE OF ADDRESS Please forward to the subscriptions address listed above 6 weeks prior to move; enclose present mailing label with change of address. POSTMASTER: send address changes to *Cancer*, Jeff Lettiere, Subscription Fulfillment and Distribution, John Wiley & Sons, Inc., 605 Third Avenue, New York, NY 10158-0012.

CLAIMS FOR MISSING ISSUES Claims for missing issues must be submitted within 6 months of the publication date.

CANCELLATIONS Subscription cancellations will not be accepted after the first issue has been mailed. Opinions expressed by the authors are their own and not necessarily those of the American Cancer Society or the publisher, John Wiley & Sons, Inc.

INDEXED BY: BIOSIS, Chemical Abstracts Service, Current Contents/Clinical Medicine, Current Contents/Life Sciences, Index Medicus/MEDLINE, Reference Update, Research Alert (ISI), Science Citation Index (ISI), SCISEARCH Database (ISI).

Printed in the United States of America. Copyright © 1998 American Cancer Society.

Introduction

Robert A. Smith, Ph.D.

Cancer Control, American Cancer Society, Atlanta, Georgia.

Lymphedema may be a side effect of breast cancer treatment, experienced by some women, that results in chronic and debilitating arm swelling. The cause of lymphedema is the destruction of the lymphatic vessels during the removal of lymph nodes under the arm, or during radiation therapy to that area after surgery. Lymphedema may be mild, moderate, or severe. It may arise immediately after treatment, or not show up for years, and for some women it is a crippling condition. For all women who suffer with lymphedema, it is a painful, daily reminder of their prior diagnosis of breast cancer. Until recently, this condition has received little attention. In order to identify the highest priority strategies for research and education, the American Cancer Society held an international conference in February 1998 in New York City. The conference, which included 60 of the world's experts, was preceded by a public forum that was attended by more than 250 breast cancer survivors, leaders of breast cancer advocacy groups, and the press. At the conclusion of the conference, recommendations for research, clinical practice, public and professional education, and advocacy were issued and are summarized in the workgroup reports that are included in these proceedings. We hope that these recommendations will accelerate progress that is already being made to reduce the risk of breast cancer treatment-related lymphedema, and better meet the needs of women who have developed lymphedema.

Funding for this workshop was made available from The Longaberger® Company's Horizon of Hope® Campaign. The Longaberger Company is a direct sales company, based in Newark, Ohio, and the largest manufacturer of hand-made, hardwood maple baskets in the United States. In 1995, The Longaberger Company entered into a program with the American Cancer Society dedicated to raising funds for breast cancer research and education through the sale of a special Horizon of Hope basket each year. Because The Longaberger Company's more than 45,000 Independent Sales Associates sell directly to customers in their homes, the annual two-month campaign provides a unique opportunity to distribute educational materials to nearly 2 million women each year about the importance of early breast cancer detection. The American Cancer Society and all those who attended this Workshop wish to express their gratitude to The Longaberger Company for their dedication to the fight against breast cancer.

Address for reprints: Robert A. Smith, Ph.D., American Cancer Society, Inc., Cancer Control Department, 1599 Clifton Road, NE, Atlanta, GA 30329.

American Cancer Society Lymphedema Workshop

Supplement to **Cancer**

Incidence of Breast Carcinoma-Related Lymphedema

Jeanne A. Petrek, M.D.
Melissa C. Heelan, B.A.

Department of Surgery, Memorial Sloan-Kettering Cancer Center, New York, New York.

BACKGROUND. Of the 2 million breast carcinoma survivors, perhaps 15–20% are living currently with posttreatment lymphedema. Along with the physical discomfort and disfigurement, patients with lymphedema also must cope with the distress derived from these symptoms.

METHODS. To review the medical literature for the question of lymphedema incidence, a comprehensive, computerized search was performed. All publications with subject headings designating breast carcinoma-related lymphedema from 1970 to the present (116 reports) were found, and each summary or abstract was read. Of the 116 reports, 35 discussed the incidence of lymphedema. Of these, seven reports since 1990 from five countries with the most relevance to current patients were then chosen for greater analysis and comparison.

RESULTS. The incidence of lymphedema ranged from 6% to 30%. The source of patients, length of follow-up, measurement techniques, and definition of lymphedema varied from report to report. In general, reports with shorter follow-up reported lower incidences of lymphedema.

CONCLUSIONS. The definitive study to determine the incidence of lymphedema has not been performed to date. There has been no prospective study in which patients have been followed at intervals with accurate measurement techniques over the long term. *Cancer* **1998;83:2776–81.** © *1998 American Cancer Society.*

KEYWORDS: breast carcinoma, lymphedema, quality of life, treatment complication.

Presented at the American Cancer Society Lymphedema Workshop, New York, New York, February 20–22, 1998.

Supported by the Department of Defense (DAMD17-J-94-4276).

Address for reprints: Jeanne A. Petrek, M.D., Department of Surgery, Memorial Sloan-Kettering Cancer Center, 1275 York Avenue, Room MRI 1026, New York, NY 10021.

Received July 2, 1998; accepted August 20, 1998.

In a recent statement to the press,[1] the director of the National Cancer Institute reported that 8.5 million Americans are living after the diagnosis of cancer, of which a large fraction, about 2 million, are breast carcinoma survivors. With such large numbers, it behooves clinicians and scientists to study the health-related quality of life after breast carcinoma treatment. Except for breast carcinoma recurrence, no event is more dreaded than the development of lymphedema.

Lymphedema is distressing. Along with the deformity, the swelling causes discomfort and disability. Recurrent episodes of cellulitis and lymphangitis may be expected. Added to the physical symptoms is the pain caused unintentionally by the clinicians who, interested in carcinoma recurrence, trivialize the nonlethal nature of lymphedema. The appearance of arm swelling is more distressing than that of a mastectomy, because the latter can be hidden easily, but the disfigured arm/hand is a constant reminder of the disease to the woman herself and a subject of curiosity to others.

Presentation

Lymphedema is the result of a functional overload of the lymphatic system in which lymph volume exceeds transport capabilities. The build-up of interstitial macromolecules leads to an increase in oncotic pressure in the tissues, producing more edema. Persistent swelling and stagnant protein eventually lead to fibrosis and provide an excellent culture medium for repeated bouts of cellulitis and lymphangitis. With dilatation of the lymphatics, the valves become incompetent, causing further stasis.

Lymphedema can begin insidiously at variable periods after axillary treatment. The swelling may range from being mild and barely noticeable, especially in the early stages, to a seriously disabling enlargement.

Lymphedema Quantitation

Various methods in the medical literature have been used to measure the lymphedematous arm. The traditional method is the comparison of the two arms with tape-measured circumference usually 10 cm below or 10 cm above either the olecranon or the lateral epicondyle. Such measurements can vary according to the degree of constriction of the soft tissues with the tape. Measurement of more than one location of the lower arm and upper arm (instead of relying on a single value) is important since the shape of the arm can differ among individuals before and after swelling as well as in the same individual. Measurement of the arm volume by water displacement is more accurate and can be used with a single value, but the technique is unwieldy and infrequently employed. Other more sophisticated methods (of little clinical use) include dichromatic differential absorptiometry[2] and computed tomography.[3] Conference papers in this supplement will discuss other techniques for quantitation.

There is no standard degree of enlargement which constitutes lymphedema. Although 2 cm difference between arms is the most common definition, such swelling could be severe in a thin arm and unnoticeable in heavy arms. Natural variation can rarely result in a 2 cm greater circumference in the dominant and asymmetrically muscled extremity.[4] Thus, for more accuracy, measurement of both arms, including preoperatively, is necessary.

Scientific Evaluation of Lymphedema

Research in all areas of lymphedema has been notably limited. Reasons for the scanty evaluation of lymphedema include 1) the prolonged course for development with a greater percentage of women developing lymphedema with longer follow-up, 2) lack of contact with the treating physicians—the original surgeon and/or the radiotherapist—and, most importantly, 3) lymphedema, with other issues concerning quality of life, has been viewed as less important than the eradication of cancer and detection of recurrence.

METHODS

A computerized search of the medical literature was undertaken. By using the search engine, MEDLINE (Ovid Technologies, Inc., New York, NY), the medical subject heading (MeSH) "lymphedema" was combined with one of three other MeSH terms: "breast cancer," "breast carcinoma," or "breast neoplasm." MEDLINE includes foreign language journals with an English summary and MeSH terms. There were 116 publications with these three MeSH term combinations found in the years from 1970 to the present (March 31, 1998).

Over the time period, there has been an absolute increase in the number of reports on breast carcinoma-related lymphedema. However, within the same time frame, there has also been an explosion of new medical journals with a consequent rise of reports on every topic, and it is not clear whether there has been any real increase relative to other scientific topics. Of the 116 total reports, there was 1 report from 1970 to 1974, 10 from 1975 to 1979, 9 from 1980 to 1984, 22 from 1985 to 1989, 38 from 1990 to 1994, and 36 from 1995 to 1997.

The authors publishing these reports were from the United States (48 reports), France (13 reports), Germany (13 reports), Japan (8 reports), and Italy (7 reports), and 27 reports were from 15 other countries.

The 116 reports were classified further according to content in the summary or abstract by the authors (see Fig. 1). There were 35 reports referring to the incidence of lymphedema. To review the question of the proportion of breast carcinoma survivors developing lymphedema, reports were chosen from the 35 reports for comparative analysis if they 1) were published since 1990, 2) defined the source of patients, 3) described the measurement methods, and 4) noted the interval of follow-up from treatment to measurement.

RESULTS
Lymphedema Incidence

From 35 possible reports, seven studies[5–11] were chosen for a comparative analysis and are displayed in Table 1. The reports of Ferrandez et al.[10] and Schunemann and Willich[11] were translated from the French and German, respectively. The other five reports[5–9] were written in the English language. Because only a few of the reports state the breast carcinoma treatment of their patient population, it was not possible to include this important variable in the comparative analysis. Nevertheless, by focussing on the more recently published reports, these seven studies should be most relevant to current patients and their treatments.

All reports on the incidence of lymphedema, including the seven chosen, are retrospective and suffer from the imprecision of the incidence of lymphedema.

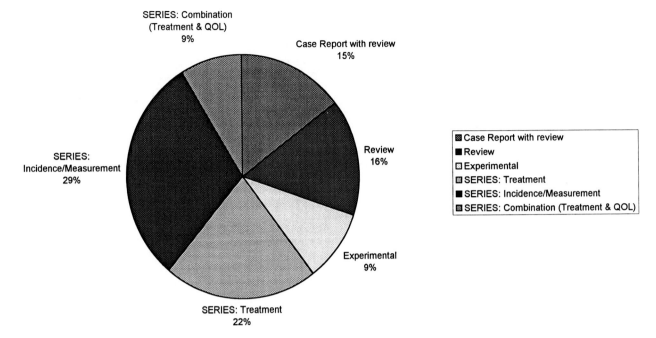

FIGURE 1. Classification of 116 medical literature reports on lymphedema between 1970 and 1997. QOL, quality of life.

TABLE 1
Seven Reports Published Since 1990 on the Incidence of Lymphedema

Yr	First author/journal	Country	Type of measurement	Definition	Incidence (%)	F/U	No. patients/source (treatment yrs)
1991	Werner/*Radiology*[5]	United States	Circumference	≥2.5 cm	19.5	37 mos[a]	282/clinic F/U (1980–1989)
1992	Ball/*Ann R Coll Surg*[6]	England	Circumference	>3 cm	6	>12 mos	50/one surgeon (1982–1990)
			Patient report	N/A	16		
1992	Ivens/*Br J Surg*[7]	England	Volumetric	>200 ml	10	2 yrs[a]	106/clinic F/U (1986–1990)
				<3 cm	16		
				3–4 cm	6		
1993	Lin/*J Clin Oncol*[8]	United States	Circumference	>4 cm	2	2 yrs[a]	283/four surgeons (1988–1990)
				≤4 cm	8.7		
				>4–8 cm	13.7		
1986	Paci/*Tumori*[9]	Italy	Circumference	≥8 cm	7.9	5 yrs[a]	238/tumor registry (1985–1986)
				>3–<10 cm	14.3		
1996	Ferrandez/*Bull Cancer*[10]	France	Circumference	≥10 cm	2.6	14 mos[a]	683/clinic F/U (1994)
1997	Schunemann/*Deutsch Med Wschr*[11]	Germany	Circumference	≥2 cm	24	11 yrs[b]	5868/clinic F/U (1972–1995)

F/U: follow-up; N/A: not available.
[a] Median time F/U.
[b] Total.

In all reports, the denominator is unknown: the number of patients at risk for developing lymphedema in that particular population.

Table 1 shows that the incidence varied from 6%[6] to 30%.[9] The reported incidence of lymphedema varies along with the methods used to define lymphedema, the source of the patients, the completeness of the patient population follow-up, and the interval between axillary treatment and measurement of lymphedema. The report with the lowest incidence of lymphedema[6] also had the shortest follow-up and included patients returning to the clinic 12 months after axillary dissection. In this series, the patients were all operated by the same surgeon—one of the authors.

In the 1960s (before the time of the computerized search used in this review), when the radical mastectomy and modified radical mastectomy were the only treatment, the incidence of lymphedema also varied greatly. In a review by American authors Britton and Nelson,[12] lymphedema incidence ranged between 6.7% and 62.5% among nine reports, and a similar review by British authors Hughes and Patel[13] found a range of 41–70% among several reports.

In the first report of Table 1,[5] 282 patients had breast conservation surgery, and all had radiation at Memorial Hospital where the report originated. Unselected patients were measured at a routine follow-up visit. The median interval between treatment and measurement was 37 months (range, 7–109). The 5-year actuarial rate of lymphedema (defined as circumference 2.5 cm larger on the treated side) was 16%.

The second report[6] notes the lowest incidence of lymphedema. Fifty patients who had surgery for breast carcinoma between 1982 and 1990 by one surgeon were examined for lymphedema when they returned for routine follow-up at least 12 months after surgery. Six percent had an arm circumference difference of greater than 3 cm between arms. All patients had a full axillary clearance in conjunction with either a wide local excision or mastectomy as well as postoperative radiotherapy to the breast or chest wall skin flaps.

In a study of 106 women at the Royal South Harts Hospital,[7] 10% of women returning for surgical follow-up were found to have lymphedema by volumetric displacement. A difference of 200 mL from the contralateral arm was defined as lymphedema. There was a median follow-up of 2 years.

In patients treated from 1988 to 1990 at Johns Hopkins University[8] on cooperative group protocols, the lymphedema incidence was 16% (defined as 2 cm circumference difference between arms) at more than 1 year after breast carcinoma treatment. With only 43% of patients returning and thereby evaluated, the lymphedema incidence may be higher, because patients may not return to the doctor associated with the complication.

From the Tumor Registry in Florence, Italy, 238 women diagnosed with breast carcinoma in 1985 and 1986 agreed to be measured out of a possible 347 who were invited to participate.[9] Lymphedema incidence was 30.2%. There were 8% who had extreme lymphedema with a difference of 8 cm between the two arms. The reason for the high incidence and severity of lymphedema is not suggested, although women with lymphedema may have been more likely to agree to become study subjects. Circumference measurements were taken at a median of 5 years after breast carcinoma surgery, making this data set one of the longer term evaluations.

In a retrospective study of 683 women in Avignon, France by Ferrandez et al.[10] the incidence of upper arm lymphedema of greater than 3 cm was 16.9%. The proportion of women developing lymphedema was the same when they were divided into mastectomy or breast conserving treatment. However, of the lymphedematous patients, the mastectomy group had a substantially greater degree of swelling.

The last report in Table 1[11] is one of the largest on posttreatment lymphedema with long follow-up. In Bad Trissl, Germany, 5868 women registered in the Oncology Clinic were evaluated for lymphedema. There were 1405 cases of arm edema (24%) at measurement, with a median follow-up of 11 years. Lymphedema was defined as having a difference of arm circumferences of greater than or equal to 2 cm. There was frequent use of postoperative radiotherapy, which was used in more than half of women who had radical mastectomy, modified radical mastectomy, or breast conserving surgery. In each of the three surgical categories, the addition of radiotherapy substantially increased the incidence of lymphedema.

DISCUSSION

These studies are retrospective, and each has relatively small numbers of patients over a long time period, often from a single institution or department. The definition of lymphedema and its measurement varied from study to study. Nevertheless, the largest flaw is knowledge of the denominator. There is incomplete information on the total number of patients at risk from lymphedema versus the number with lymphedema; therefore, the incidence stated is imprecise.

Authors' Data

The definitive study on lymphedema would include a large population of consecutive patients with data acquired prospectively on multiple patient characteristics and treatment variables, accurate arm measurements preoperatively and at intervals during follow-up, data on suspected causative factors in subsequent years (such as arm infections), and minimal proportion lost to follow-up in a long term study. Knowing all of the rigid criteria for a definitive study, especially the several years of interval measurements and thereby the expense, the authors examined available hospital data sets for the possibility of useful information that could be obtained at present. With a grant from the federal government (DAMA 17-J-94-4276), a study on lymphedema was performed on a research patient cohort at Memorial Sloan-Kettering Cancer Center.

A preexisting research data set of 1216 consecutively treated patients at Memorial Sloan-Kettering

Cancer Center from 1976 to 1978 was used. Only 2% of the women diagnosed and treated during that time period were not entered. Patient characteristics and treatment variables were obtained prospectively. The cohort has been followed annually, with interval medical history for breast carcinoma recurrence and overall survival. Multiple funded research projects and publications have resulted: Obesity at diagnosis as a prognostic factor,[14] the effect of histologic variables on outcome,[15] risk of multicentricity and bilaterality,[16] and others.[17–19] However, before the present research project, nowhere in the 18–20 year course of follow-up were they assessed for lymphedema.

In 1997, various endpoints related to lymphedema and its suspected etiologic factors were assessed by the same research nurse in these patients. Self reported arm circumference measurements at two sites also were obtained by using a method validated on nonprotocol patients.

There were 336 women living in 1996 (only 42 patients had been lost to follow-up). Of these 336 women, 64 were unable (medical reasons) or refused to participate, and 272 women were study subjects on whom complete data and circumferential measurements were obtained. Of 272 study patients, 32 (12%) had enlargement of 2 inches or more in circumference over the contralateral arm that was designated as severe lymphedema. If those with some measurable enlargement, but less than 2 inches, are included, then an additional 43 women had lymphedema. About half of the patients with documented minimal enlargement (1–2 cm) suffer symptoms of "arm heaviness."[20]

Based on these two categories, 75 of 272 patients (28%) have measurable lymphedema. Another 47 of 272 patients (17%) also stated in the research interview that their arm "felt" swollen. In the last category, there was no measurable difference, and they had not seen a medical professional for lymphedema. In another population of patients, a survey found that half of the patients acknowledging arm swelling in a mail questionnaire had never reported this problem to any doctor or other health care provider.[21] An unknown proportion of breast carcinoma survivors may indeed have slight but unmeasurable lymphedema. Because that may be the case in these study patients, they are included in the "all" lymphedema category in the effort to be inclusive. To evaluate etiologic factors, the data were analyzed with all levels of lymphedema, with the two measurable levels and with severe lymphedema alone, and the results are undergoing statistical analysis.

Surprisingly, the treatment of a contralateral breast carcinoma was not associated with a higher incidence of lymphedema. Of the 272 women, 55 women were treated for contralateral breast carcinoma and had a lower incidence of lymphedema in the index arm (not significant) than those who received unilateral breast carcinoma treatment. Another large data set with contralateral breast carcinoma had similar findings.[22]

CONCLUSIONS

In sum, objective lymphedema incidence in seven reports published in 1990, as noted in Table 1, was about 20%.[5–11] The range was 6%[6] to 30%[9] of the diverse study populations measured at various intervals after axillary dissection with arm circumferences or volumetric equipment. Table 1 is comprised of patients who underwent different surgical and radiotherapeutic procedures for breast carcinoma treatment in the United States, England, Italy, France, and Germany. In general, these reports show higher incidence and more severe swelling related to longer follow-up. However, in the reports with longer follow-up, more extensive breast carcinoma treatment was the standard in those years, and the treatment factor also may contribute to a higher risk of lymphedema.

The incidence of lymphedema seems to be decreasing in more modern times, according to practicing surgeons. This is probably due to earlier diagnosis of less advanced breast carcinomas that can be treated with lesser axillary procedures. In turn, this trend seems to be due to mammographic screening and public education efforts. Furthermore, the development of two modern techniques—sentinel lymph node biopsy technology, allowing less axillary surgery and more precise radiation planning, and delivery, allowing less radiation to the axilla—should also contribute to the decrease in the incidence of lymphedema.

REFERENCES

1. Stolberg SG. New cancer cases decreasing in U.S. as deaths do, too. *New York Times* March 13, 1998.
2. Bolin FP, Preuss LE, Beninson J. Di-chromatic differential absorptiometry for assessment of lymphedema. *Int J Nucl Med Biol* 1980;7:449–51.
3. Stewart G, Hurst PAE, Thomas ML, Burnand KG. CAT scanning in the management of the lymphedematous limb. *Immunol Hematol Res* 1988;2:241–24.
4. Kissin MW, Querci della Rovere G, Easton D, Westburg G. Risk of lymphoedema following the treatment of breast cancer. *Br J Surg* 1986;73:580–4.
5. Werner RS, McCormick B, Petrek JA, Cox L, Cirrincione C, Gray JR, et al. Arm edema in conservatively managed breast cancer: obesity is a major predictive factor. *Ther Radiol* 1991;180:177–84.
6. Ball ABS, Fish S, Waters R, Meirion Thomas J. Radical axillary dissection in the staging and treatment of breast cancer. *Ann R Coll Surg Engl* 1992;74:126–9.

7. Ivens D, Hoe AL, Podd CR, Hamilton CR, Taylor I, Royle GT. Assessment of morbidity from complete axillary dissection. *Br J Cancer* 1992;66:136–8.

8. Lin PP, Allison DC, Wainstock J, Miller KD, Dooley WC, Friedman N. Impact of axillary lymph node dissection on the therapy of breast cancer patients. *J Clin Oncol* 1993; 11(8):1536–44.

9. Paci E, Cariddi A, Barchielli A, Bianchi S, Cardona G, Distante V, et al. Long-term sequelae of breast cancer surgery. *Tumori* 1996;82:321–4.

10. Ferrandez JC, Serin D, Bouges S. Frequence des lymphoedemes du membre superieur apres traitement du cancer du sein. Facteurs de risque. A propos de 683 observations. *Bull Cancer* 1996;83:989–95.

11. Schunemann H, Willich N. Lymphodeme nach mammakarzinom. Eine studie uber 5868 falle. *Deutsch Med Wschr* 1997;122:536–41.

12. Britton RC, Nelson PA. Causes and treatment of post-mastectomy lymphedema of the arm. Report of 114 cases. *JAMA* 1962;180:95–102.

13. Hughes JH, Patel AR. Swelling of the arm following radical mastectomy. *Br J Surg* 1966;53:4–14.

14. Senie RT, Rosen PP, Rhodes P, Lesser ML, Kinne DW. Obesity at diagnosis of breast carcinoma influences duration of disease-free survival. *Ann Intern Med* 1992;116:26–32.

15. Rosen PP, Lesser ML, Senie RL, Kinne DW. Epidemiology of breast carcinoma III: relationship of family history to tumor type. *Cancer* 1982;50:171–9.

16. Lesser ML, Rosen PP, Kinne DW. Multicentricity and bilaterality of invasive breast carcinoma. *Surgery* 1982;91:234–40.

17. Senie RT, Rosen PP, Lesser ML, Snyder RE, Schottenfeld D, Duthie K. Epidemiology of breast carcinoma II: factors related to the predominance of left-sided disease. *Cancer* 1980;46:1705–13.

18. Senie RT, Rosen PP, Lesser ML, Kinne DW. Breast self-examination and medical examination related to breast cancer stage. *Am J Public Health* 1981;71:583–90.

19. Senie RT, Lobenthal SW, Rosen PP. Association of vaginal smear cytology with menstrual status in breast cancer. *Breast Cancer Res Treat* 1985;5:301–10.

20. Brennan MJ. Lymphedema following the surgical treatment of breast cancer: a review of pathophysiology and treatment. *J Pain Symp Manage* 1992;7:110–6.

21. McCaffrey JF. Lymphedema–Its treatment In: Fundamental problems in breast cancer. Paterson AHG, Lees AW, editors. Boston: Martinus Nijhoff Publishing, 1987:259–63.

22. Mortimer PS, Bates DO, Brassington HD, Stanton AWB, Strachan DP, Levick JR. The prevalence of arm oedema following treatment for breast cancer. *Q J Med* 1996;89: 377–80.

Surgical Treatment and Lymphedema

Peter I. Pressman, M.D.

Department of Surgery, Albert Einstein College of Medicine, New York, New York.

Department of Surgery, Beth Israel Medical Center and Lenox Hill Hospital, New York, New York.

BACKGROUND. Lymphedema is a serious and disabling complication of the treatment of breast carcinoma. This is related directly to the removal of axillary lymph nodes. Because lymph node status is the single most important predictor of outcome, it is necessary to obtain accurate information. Whereas breast conservation has become the preferred approach for treating early breast carcinoma, the accompanying axillary dissection continues to cause morbidity.

METHODS. The history of the operations for breast carcinoma is reviewed, and the anatomy, techniques, and complications of axillary lymphadenectomy are described. Data to support the necessity for accurate axillary staging is presented, and results of noninvasive axillary staging approaches are discussed. The technique and value of sentinel node biopsy are presented.

RESULTS. Axillary lymphadenectomy is required where lymph node metastases are present to accomplish local control, improve survival, and provide information for staging to plan adjunctive therapy. Noninvasive techniques do not yet provide high enough sensitivity to assess the status of the axilla. The sentinel lymph node biopsy is a technique that can identify those patients who require axillary lymphadenectomy.

CONCLUSIONS. Screening mammography has been responsible for down-staging the size of detected breast carcinomas, so that the axillary dissection may be omitted in small carcinomas of favorable histologic type. For carcinomas in which the probability of axillary metastases exists, by using the sentinel lymph node biopsy, axillary dissections can be avoided when results are negative, and the risk of lymphedema can be reduced. *Cancer* **1998;83:2782–7.**
© *1998 American Cancer Society.*

KEYWORDS: axilla, breast carcinoma, lymphadenectomy, sentinel node biopsy.

Presented at the American Cancer Society Lymphedema Workshop, New York, New York, February 20–22, 1998.

Dr. Pressman is Clinical Professor of Surgery at the Albert Einstein College of Medicine and is an Attending Surgeon at Beth Israel Medical Center and Lenox Hill Hospital.

Address for reprints: Peter I. Pressman, M.D., 787 Park Avenue, New York, NY 10021.

Received July 2, 1998; accepted August 20, 1998.

The removal of axillary lymph nodes has been an integral part of breast carcinoma treatment since the end of the last century. The earliest approaches to control breast carcinoma were simple tumor excisions, and these did not work. To avoid the certainty of local recurrence and the sequelae of ulceration, bleeding, infection, and pain, a much wider removal of tissues was required. Even the complete mastectomy needed to be enlarged to include the muscles of the chest wall, frequently because of direct invasion of the locally advanced malignancies being treated. In the evolution of the understanding of the behavior of breast carcinoma, the necessity to remove the axillary lymph nodes was based on both clinical and pathologic observation. The radical mastectomy, introduced in the late 1800s, accomplished the goal of decreasing local recurrence; and longer survival, not anticipated previously, became a reality. Many of those women had advanced breast carcinomas that would be considered inoperable today; thus, these results were remarkable. Removal of diseased lymph nodes was important.[1]

Breast carcinoma treatment continued to evolve during this century. There were attempts to improve the outcome of the Halsted radical mastectomy by enlarging the operation to include supraclavicular and the internal mammary lymph nodes[2] and by extending the radical mastectomy to include en bloc resection of the internal mammary lymph nodes with the chest wall.[3] However, no survival advantage could be demonstrated for these superradical procedures.[4] The modified radical mastectomy supplanted the more radical procedures in the 1970s, and, in turn, was followed a decade later by breast conservation using limited resections and radiation therapy. For women now who need to have a breast removed, reconstruction usually can be carried out at the same time. Implants can be used, and myocutaneous flaps, such as the transrectus ambominus muscle (TRAM), can create such natural looking results that women do not appear to have had a mastectomy at all.

Breast Carcinoma Behavior

The behavior of breast carcinoma is characterized by a tendency to recur locally and also to spread by vascular and lymphatic pathways. Successful treatment necessitates both obtaining local control and addressing the risk of systemic dissemination. The initial interpretation credited to Halsted was that there was a predictable scenario: that carcinoma originated in the breast and spread in a contiguous manner by direct extension and through lymphatics to the lymph nodes and then to distant sites. This theory was challenged by those who interpreted breast carcinoma always as a systemic disease from inception and considered the treatment of lymph nodes to be less important.[5,6] In fact, there appear to be different patterns of behavior. Some breast carcinomas never spread to the axillary lymph nodes but disseminate early through the blood stream, whereas other carcinomas may metastasize even extensively to the axillary lymph nodes, which, when removed, results in disease free survival for the patient.[7] Treatment strategies are based on these theories.

The Removal of Axillary Lymph Nodes

Axillary lymph nodes are removed to provide accurate information for staging, to accomplish local control, and for prognosis in order to plan adjunctive, systemic therapy. The status of the axillary lymph nodes remains the single most important predictor of survival.[8,9] It is because of the morbidity associated with the procedure that questions have been raised about its necessity, particularly in treating the smaller breast carcinomas that are detected today.

Morbidity of Axillary Lymphadenectomy

- Seroma formation
- Discomfort
- Numbness
- Limitation of shoulder movement
- Lymphedema (arm)
- Breast edema.

Some of the secondary effects of axillary dissection are acute and transient; however, lymphedema is the most serious and is a continuing complication. The incidence varies according to the diligence used in measuring the arm and the length of patient follow-up.[10] Although there are probably many factors that influence the development of lymphedema, if the axillary lymph nodes are not removed, then lymphedema does not occur. Where the surgical dissection is more extensive, or if radiation therapy is used postoperatively to treat the axilla and adjacent lymphatics, then the probability of subsequently developing lymphedema increases.

The Axillary Dissection

The evolution toward breast conservation has been accompanied by a less radical approach to the axillary dissection. The first modification of the radical mastectomy described by Patey was called the conservative radical. Preserving the pectoralis major muscle improved the cosmetic appearance, and this was an important advance, however, the pectoralis minor muscle was excised specifically to facilitate a similar radical axillary lymph node clearance.[11] In 1963, Auchincloss demonstrated that an equivalent rate of cure could be obtained by saving the pectoralis minor muscle and not dissecting the highest level of the axilla. He called this operation a simple mastectomy and subtotal axillary dissection and employed it for carcinoma in situ. This conservatism was justified, because, except in patients with extensive axillary metastases, removing nodes at levels I and II was adequate.[12]

Anatomy of the Axilla

The axillary lymph nodes at the tail of the breast are surrounded by fat, and this is level I. The anatomic boundaries are the axillary vein superiorly, the latissimus dorsi muscle laterally, the subscapular vessels and the thoracodorsal nerve posteriorly, and the lateral border of the pectoralis minor muscle and the long thoracic nerve medially (Fig. 1).

Lymph nodes posterior to the pectoralis minor muscle are designated as level II. Separation between these levels is not at all exact, because retraction of the pectoral muscles in the course of the operative procedure for exposure obscures any separation between

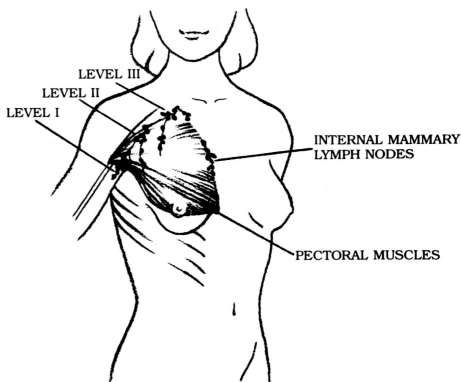

FIGURE 1. Diagram of axilla (reprinted with permission from Y. Hirshaut and P. Pressman[13]).

these levels. Only if these lymph nodes are labeled by the surgeon after removal can they be identified according to level by the pathologist.

Level III is medial to the pectoralis minor muscle at the chest wall, and this is the apex of the axilla. There are additional lymph nodes between the pectoral muscles (Rotter's nodes) and overlying the axillary vein, along the subscapular vessels and the thoracodorsal nerve, and scattered over the chest wall.

Over the decades, the modified radical has become a more modest operation. Skin grafting is a procedure of the past. Larger amounts of skin and subcutaneous tissues are retained and used for breast reconstruction. The pectoralis minor muscle is removed rarely, so that level III lymph nodes rarely are excised. Rotter's nodes, the lymphatic tissue between the pectoral muscles, usually are not dissected. Formerly, the axillary dissection implied skeletonizing the axillary vein and clearing the fascial covering of the chest wall muscles overlying the ribs. The total number of lymph nodes removed by axillary dissection has decreased with the less extensive operations currently being performed. Currently, most women with Stage I and II breast carcinoma are able to conserve their breasts with the use of radiation therapy following tumorectomy. Lymph node dissection remains an integral part of this approach but has become more minimal, because, when the breast is treated postop-

eratively with radiation, so are the subjacent tissues of the low axilla.[14]

Local Control

Recurrence in the axilla not only is disappointing for patients but is associated with a poor prognosis, may be difficult to manage surgically, and is a cause of lymphedema following secondary treatment. The NSABP B-04 study has been the most frequently cited study showing evidence that dissection of the clinically negative axilla is diagnostic and does not have therapeutic value.[15] However, there has been evidence that inadequate treatment of lymph nodes impacts adversely on survival[16,17] and that prophylactic dissection of the clinically negative axilla does improve survival.[18] This is the therapeutic reason for removing lymph nodes.

Staging

The presence or absence of lymph node metastases remains the single most important predictor of outcome, even with the multiple prognostic factors that have been developed.[8,9] Accurate information is vital for staging and for making decisions about systemic therapy and is required for patients in clinical trials to assess treatment outcome intelligently. Because systemic adjuvant chemotherapy and tamoxifen improve survival, it is recommended where lymph nodes are negative.[19] However, with tumors of smaller size (T1a–T1b; 1 cm), the presence of lymph node metastases can be the decisive factor governing a recommendation for systemic therapy.[20]

Prognostic Value

Surgeons always have been sensitive to the potential for lymphedema subsequent to axillary lymph node dissections and have investigated other means for predicting axillary node involvement. Clinical palpation of the axilla is inaccurate in assessing lymph node status. Approximately 35% of the time, a clinically negative axilla will contain positive lymph nodes.[21,22] Intraoperative, random sampling of lymph nodes has not proven to be accurate.[23] However, the predictive value of a complete level I and II dissection is very high. If this is negative, then the chance that there are metastases at higher levels is negligible.[24]

Sentinel Lymphadenectomy

A potential alternative to axillary dissections is the sentinel node biopsy. This is a technique of intraoperative lymphatic mapping in which either a blue dye (lymphazurin)[25] or a radioactive colloid[26] is injected into the breast around the carcinoma. After a planned time interval, the axilla is explored through a surgical incision, and the lymphatics are followed to the first lymph node, which picks up the dye or isotope. This is called the sentinel node. If this lymph node contains no malignancy, then it predicts for the negativity of the axilla, and a formal lymph node dissection can be avoided. If a metastasis is found either on the initial frozen section examination or on subsequent examination of the lymph node, which includes conventional hematoxylin and eosin staining and immunohistochemical examination, then the axillary dissection is completed. This procedure requires experience, so that, ideally, a false negative rate of less than 3% can be obtained. It is most successful when the dye or isotope can be injected around an undisturbed primary carcinoma. This requires a preliminary needle biopsy to establish the diagnosis of malignancy; therefore, it necessitates some changes in current surgical practice. For many women and for certain pathologies, it has been desirable to perform an initial, separate, excisional biopsy; to review and discuss the findings; and to make informed decisions about treatment options. The biopsied breast is not as amenable to accurate sentinel node biopsy. Multicentric or large tumors also are not mapped as accurately as small carcinomas. It is not advised for patients with clinically positive axillary lymph nodes. Patients have not yet been followed long enough to know whether lymphedema will occur and whether this procedure

will result in under staging and omitting of systemic therapy where it may be important. Sentinel node biopsy is a major advance and needs to be integrated into our surgical armamentarium. It has the potential for decreasing the numbers of axillary dissections.[27]

Noninvasive Axillary Staging

It would be ideal if the status of the axillary lymph nodes could be predicted with a noninvasive approach. One technique being investigated is radioimmunoscintography. A technectium-labeled monoclonal antibody is injected intravenously, and the axilla is scanned. Lymph nodes containing metastases can be identified with a sensitivity reported as 90% and a specificity of 85%.[28] Another technique is positron emission tomography (PET) scanning of the axilla, with a reported sensitivity of 72% and a specificity of 96%.[29] False negative PET findings occur mainly with micrometastases; therefore, these techniques are investigative and are not yet accurate enough to substitute for surgical evaluation of the axilla.[30]

Omitting the Axillary Dissection

Selecting certain carcinomas in which removing axillary lymph nodes can be omitted is a desirable goal. Routine axillary lymph node dissection has been eliminated for ductal carcinoma in situ, because the risk of axillary metastases is under 1%.[31] Microinvasive carcinoma[32] and pure tubular carcinomas under 1 cm[33] and medullary and mucinous carcinomas also have an extremely low risk of axillary metastases.[34] These are rare lesions. The probability of axillary lymph node metastases (ALNM) does increase as a function of tumor size. In 918 patients with T1 tumors recently reported by Silverstein et al.,[30] the incidence of ALNM was 23%. Four factors were identified as predictors of ALNM: tumor size, tumor palpability, nuclear grade, and lymphovascular invasion. Where all four factors were favorable—under 1 cm (T1a–b), nonpalpable tumors, low nuclear grade, and without lymph/vascular invasion—there was a 3% incidence of ALNM.[35] These patients may be spared an axillary dissection.

Early Detection

Because of the widespread use of mammography over the past 25 years, an increasing percentage of carcinomas are being detected and treated at the in situ stage for which an axillary dissection is not needed. Cady has emphasized that there has been a progressive decrease in the greatest dimension of breast carcinomas (Fig. 2). Mammographically detected carcinomas have a lesser incidence of nodal involvement, particularly those less than 1 cm (T1a and T1b).[36] It is possible, particularly in discussion and with the par-

Size of Invasive Breast Cancer- NEDH

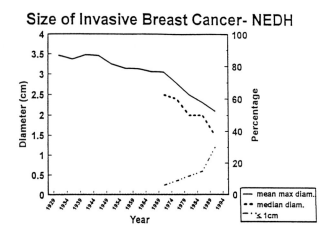

FIGURE 2. Mean and median (when calculated) maximum dimensions (in cm) and proportion of cases measuring 1 cm or less in maximum dimension (T1a and T1b) in all invasive breast carcinomas of Stages I, II, and III at the New England Deaconess Hospital (Boston, MA), over time (reprinted with permission from B. Cady[35]).

ticipation of informed patients, to omit the axillary dissection or perform a sentinel node biopsy in those cases in which the likelihood of lymph node involvement is very low.

The guidelines for screening with mammography have been recommended by both the American Cancer Society and the National Cancer Institute.[37] Screening is responsible for down-staging—finding more curable carcinomas that require less treatment and result in better survival. Because of programs of early detection and particularly the widespread use of mammography, most women with breast carcinoma today are being treated at an earlier stage of disease. This has resulted in more breast conservation and has started to contribute to a decline in mortality.[38] The best approach to preventing lymphedema is to limit the necessity for the surgical removal of axillary lymph nodes. The potential currently exists to accomplish this goal.

REFERENCES

1. Halsted WS. The result of operations for the cure of cancer of the breast. *Ann Surg* 1907;46:1–9.
2. Dalh-Iversen E, Tobiassen T. Radical mastectomy with parasternal and supraclavicular dissection for mammary carcinoma. *Ann Surg* 1963;157:170–5.
3. Urban JA. Radical excision of the chest wall for mammary cancer. *Cancer* 1951;4:263–85.
4. Veronesi U, Valagussa P. Inefficacy of internal mammary nodes dissection in breast cancer surgery. *Cancer* 1981;47:170–5.
5. Fisher B, Montague E. Comparison of radical mastectomy with alternative treatments for primary breast cancer. *Cancer* 1977;39:2829–39.
6. Fisher B. Laboratory and clinical research in breast cancer—a personal adventure: The David Karnovsky Memorial Lecture. *Cancer Res* 1980;40:3863–74.
7. Hellman S. Natural history of small breast cancers. *J Clin Oncol* 1994;12:2229–34.
8. Fisher B, Bauer M, Margolese R, Poisson R, Pilch Y, Redmond C, et al. Five-year results of a randomized clinical trial comparing total mastectomy and segmental mastectomy with or without radiation in the treatment of breast cancer. *N Engl J Med* 1985;312:665–73.
9. Mustafa I, Bland K. Indications for axillary dissection in T1 breast cancer. *Ann Surg* 1998;5:4–8.
10. Petrak JA, Blackwood MM. Axillary dissection: current practice and technique. *Curr Probl Surg* 1995;32:312–4.
11. Patey DH, Dyson WH. Prognosis of carcinoma of the breast in relation to type of operation performed. *Br J Cancer* 1948;2:7–12.
12. Auchincloss H. Significance of location and number of axillary metastases in carcinoma of the breast. *Ann Surg* 1963;158(1):37–46.
13. Hirshaut Y, Pressman P. Breast cancer—the complete guide. New York: Bantam Books, 1996:114.
14. Recht A, Houlihan MJ. Axillary lymph nodes and cancer. *Cancer* 1995;76:1491–512.
15. Fisher B, Redmond C, Fisher ER, Bauer M, Wolmark N, Wickerham DL, et al. Ten-year results of a randomized clinical trial comparing radical mastectomy and total mastectomy with or without radiation. *N Engl J Med* 1985;312:674–81.
16. Cabanes PA, Salmon RJ, Vilcoq JR, Durand JC, Fourquet A, Gautier C, Asselain B. Value of axillary dissection in addition to lumpectomy and radiotherapy in early breast cancer. *Lancet* 1992;339:1245–8.
17. Harris JR, Osteen RT. Patients with early breast cancer benefit from effective axillary treatment. *Breast Cancer Res Treat* 1985;5:17–21.
18. Orr R. The impact of prophylactic axillary node dissection on breast cancer survival—a Bayesian meta-analysis [abstract]. Proc Soc Surg Oncol. San Diego, CA. March 26–29, 1998.
19. Early Breast Cancer Trialist's Cooperative Group. Systemic treatment for early breast cancer by hormonal, cytotoxic or immune therapy: 133 randomized trials involving 31,000 recurrences and 24,000 deaths among 75,000 women. *Lancet* 1992;339:71–85.
20. Lin PP, Allison DC, Wainstock J, Miller KD, Dooley WC, Friedman N, Baker RR. Impact of axillary lymph node dissection on the therapy of breast cancer patient. *J Clin Oncol* 1993;11:1536–44.
21. isher B, Wolmark N, Bauer M, Redmond C, Gebhardt, M. The accuracy of clinical nodal staging and of limited axillary dissection as a determinant of histological nodal status in carcinoma of the breast. *Surg Gynecol Obstet* 1981;152:765–72.
22. Danforth D, Findlay P, McDonald H. Complete axillary lymph nodes dissection for Stage I–II carcinoma of the breast. *J Clin Oncol* 1986;4:655–62.
23. Kissin MW, Thompson EM, Price AB, Slavin G, Kark AE. The inadequacy of axillary sampling in breast cancer. *Lancet* 1982;1:1210–2.
24. Veronesi U, Rilke F, Luini A, Sacchini V, Galimberti V, Campa T, et al. Distribution of axillary nodes metastases by level of invasion: an analysis of 539 cases. *Cancer* 1987;59:682–7.
25. Giuliano AE, Kirgan DM, Guenther JM, Morton DL. Lymphatic mapping and sentinel lymphadenectomy for breast cancer. *Ann Surg* 1994;222:394–401.

26. Krag DN, Weaver DL, Alex JC, Fairbank JT. Surgical resection and radiolocalization of the sentinel lymph node in breast cancer using a gamma probe. *Surg Oncol* 1993;2:335–40.

27. Giuliano A, Jones R, Brennan M, Statman R. S=entinel lymphadenectomy in breast cancer. *J Clin Oncol* 1997;15:2345–50.

28. Biassoni L, Granowska M, Carroll MJ, Mather SJ, Howell R, Ellison D, et al. 99m Tc-labelled SM3 in the preoperative evaluation of axillary lymph nodes and primary breast cancer with change detection statistical processing as an aid to tumour detection. *Br J Cancer* 1998;77:131–8.

29. Avril N, Janicke F, Dose J, Zeigler S, Bense S, Zincke M, et al. Evaluation of axillary lymph node involvement in breast cancer patients using F-18 FDG PET. *Eur J Nucl Med* 1995;22:733–40.

30. Crippa F, Agresti R, Seregni E, Greco M, Pascali C, Bogni A, et al. Prospective evaluation of Flourine-19-FDG Pet in pre-surgical staging of the axilla in breast cancer. *J Nucl Med* 1998;39:4–8.

31. Silverstein MJ, Rosser RJ, Gierson ED, Waisman JR, Gamagami P, Hoffman RS. Axillary lymph node dissection for intraductal carcinoma: is it indicated? *Cancer* 1987;59:1819–24.

32. Silver S, Tavassoli FA. Mammary ductal carcinoma in situ with microinvasion. *Cancer* 1998(in press).

33. McDivitt RW, Boyce W, Gersell D. Tubular carcinoma of the breast: clinical and pathological observations concerning 135 cases. *Am J Surg Pathol* 1982;6:401–11.

34. Rosen PP, Groshen S, Kinne DW, Norton L. Factors influencing prognosis in node-negative breast carcinoma: analysis of 767 $T_1N_0M_0/T_2N_0M_0$ patients with long term follow-up. *J Clin Oncol* 1993;11:2090–100.

35. Barth A, Craig P, Silverstein MJ. Predictors of axillary lymph node metastases in patients with T1 breast carcinoma. *Cancer* 1997;79:1918–22.

36. Cady B. The new era in breast cancer. *Arch Surg* 1996;131:301–8.

37. Leitch AM, Dodd GD, Costanza M. American Cancer Society guidelines for the early detection of breast cancer update 1997. *Cancer* 1997;47:150–3.

38. Office of Cancer Communications. Cancer death rate declined for the first time ever in the 90s [press release, November 14, 1996]. Bethesda, MD: National Cancer Institute, 1996.

Breast Radiotherapy and Lymphedema

Allen G. Meek, M.D.

Department of Radiation Oncology, University Medical Center, Stony Brook, New York.

BACKGROUND. Breast radiotherapy has a low incidence of long term complications. Lymphedema is the most commonly reported complication and adversely affects the quality of life of the breast carcinoma patient. Although its incidence is decreasing, lymphedema still remains a significant concern for patients and their physicians. With the indications for radiotherapy in breast carcinoma management broadening, current strategies to prevent radiation-related lymphedema should be applied and new strategies should be developed.

METHODS. A review of the literature addressing lymphedema as a complication of radiotherapy in breast carcinoma management was performed.

RESULTS. Arm, breast, and truncal edema occur after primary breast carcinoma management. The literature supports the view that radiotherapy contributes to arm and breast edema. Lymphedema occurs most commonly in patients who have both axillary radiotherapy and surgery, is often triggered by a soft tissue infection, and is more common in obese patients. The incidence of arm edema is decreasing due to more conservative surgical treatment of the axilla and possibly due to more conservative management of the breast. Trends in breast edema are less discernible. Single-modality treatment of the axilla is associated with a very low incidence of arm edema.

CONCLUSIONS. Lymphedema continues to be a problem in the care of the breast carcinoma patient. More conservative surgery combined with careful patient selection for nodal radiotherapy reduces its incidence. Radiotherapy technique, prompt treatment of soft tissue infections, and weight loss in obese patients each can contribute to prevention. The risk of lymphedema is greatly surpassed by the benefits of radiotherapy in the care of the breast carcinoma patient. *Cancer* **1998; 83:2788–97.** © *1998 American Cancer Society.*

KEYWORDS: breast cancer, axilla, radiotherapy, lymphedema, soft tissue infection, obesity.

Lymphedema consequent to carcinoma management remains a major quality of life concern for the breast carcinoma patient.[1–6] Lymphedema may involve the arm, the trunk, or the conserved breast. The incidence and severity of lymphedema is related predominantly to the extent of axillary surgery but is strongly affected by added axillary radiotherapy.[2] Lymphedema virtually could be avoided completely by not dissecting or radiating the axilla.[7,8] However, axillary treatment surgically and/or with radiotherapy is still an essential component in the management of most patients with invasive breast carcinoma.[9,10] Strategies to reduce the risk of lymphedema are available to radiation oncologists so that the improved carcinoma outcomes seen with axillary treatment are not compromised by substantially worse quality of life outcomes.

In this article, the literature on breast radiotherapy is analyzed particularly with respect to the development of lymphedema. The types of lymphedema seen and their risk relative to surgical and radiation techniques are summarized. The pathophysiology of and

Presented in part at the American Cancer Society Lymphedema Workshop, New York, New York, February 20–22, 1998.

Address for reprints: Allen G. Meek, M.D., Department of Radiation Oncology, University Medical Center, Stony Brook, NY 11794-7028.

Received July 2, 1998; accepted August 20, 1998.

TABLE 1
Incidence of Lymphedema as a Function of Surgery and Axillary Radiotherapy[a]

Surgery type	Radical mastectomy (%)	Modified radical (%)	Breast conservation (%)
No radiotherapy	22	19	7
Radiotherapy	44	29	10 (RT to breast only)

RT: radiotherapy.
[a] Schunemann and Willich, 1997.[13]

patient risk factors for lymphedema also are reviewed. These risks are then synthesized with recommendations for prevention. The benefits of breast radiotherapy also are summarized briefly.

Types of Lymphedema Seen in Breast Carcinoma Patients

Three types of lymphedema are described in breast carcinoma patients: arm, truncal, and, in conservation patients, breast lymphedema. Arm lymphedema is the most commonly described[2] and feared, although breast lymphedema is the more frequent complication in breast conservation patients.[11] Reports from different institutions regarding these complications are difficult to compare due to a lack of standard measuring and reporting criteria.[2] Truncal edema, particularly affecting the posterior axillary fold, is an infrequently reported complication[12] and, because there is no reported association with radiotherapy, is not discussed further in this paper.

Contribution of Radiotherapy to Lymphedema in Breast Carcinoma Patients
Arm lymphedema
The development of arm lymphedema after breast surgery and radiotherapy is a function of the extent of

the axillary surgery,[13,14] the breast surgery,[2,13] and whether the axilla is irradiated[8,13,15] (the relative contribution of each is probably in descending order as listed). This is demonstrated by a recently reported retrospective series from Germany of almost 6000 patients treated over 23 years with over 1400 cases of lymphedema (≥ 2 cm difference in arm circumference). This study noted a decline in lymphedema over time coincident with the transition to more breast conservative surgical procedures (Table 1) and omission of axillary radiotherapy in the breast conservation group.[13] In each group of patients treated by radical mastectomy, modified radical mastectomy, or breast conservation, added radiotherapy (including the axilla in the mastectomy groups) increased the risk of lymphedema.

Clinical trials also suggest that the extent of surgical dissection is probably the greatest predictor for lymphedema risk in patients treated by mastectomy. For example, a clinical trial reported from Scotland in 1971 noted a 10% risk of arm lymphedema (≥ 3 cm difference in arm circumference) in patients treated with radical mastectomy compared with a 5% risk in patients treated with simple mastectomy and radiotherapy to the chest wall and axilla.[16] However, added radiotherapy certainly increases the risk, particularly if it is hypofractionated.[15,17] For example, in the Stockholm randomized series reported in 1981, modified radical mastectomy had a lymphedema (>10% increase in arm volume) complication rate of 10%, which increased to 16% or 18%, respectively, with preoperative or postoperative radiotherapy that included the axilla.[18] In contrast, the 1997 report of the randomized series from Vancouver noted a lymphedema (not defined) incidence of 3% in patients treated with a modified radical mastectomy without radiotherapy that increased to 9% when postoperative ra-

TABLE 2
Incidence of Arm Lymphedema in Patients Treated with Breast Radiotherapy as a Function of Axillary Treatment

Axillary treatment	None (%)	Dissection (%)	Radiotherapy (%)	Both (%)
Northwestern University[7]	0	14 (Limited) 27 (Full)		
Universitat Munster[13]		10		
University of Miami[20]		14		30 (Full dissection)
Harvard University[22,28]		3	4	13 (Average) 37 (Full dissection)
European combined[23]	0	2	2	9
Institut Curie[24]		2	2	
Hopital Henri Mondor[25]			4	25
Centre de Charlebourg[26]			3	25
Hopital Tenon[26]			3	12
Institut Gustave-Roussy[30]		2		20

diotherapy (including the axilla) was administered,[19] suggesting that added radiotherapy was a greater contributor to the risk of lymphedema.

The risk of lymphedema as a function of the extent of axillary dissection in patients not receiving axillary radiotherapy is somewhat controversial.[2] Axillary sampling alone is reported to have little to no risk of lymphedema.[8] Partial or total axillary lymphadenectomy carries a risk of up to 22% of lymphedema, with a trend, although it is not consistent, of higher risk with the more aggressive surgery.[7,8,13,20,21] The different mix of patient stages and varying definitions of axillary dissection techniques confounds the comparisons between series.

The risk of lymphedema as a function of the extent of axillary dissection in patients receiving axillary radiotherapy follows a similar pattern. Axillary sampling plus radiotherapy is associated with a 6–9% risk of lymphedema.[8,11] Partial or total axillary lymphadenectomy plus radiotherapy is associated with a 9–44% risk of lymphedema,[8,13,19–22] with a trend toward less risk in the patients who receive less aggressive axillary surgery.

The risk of lymphedema in patients receiving breast radiotherapy also depends on whether the axilla is dissected or radiated (Table 2). Most of the randomized trials comparing breast conservation plus radiotherapy versus mastectomy did not include radiotherapy to the axilla, whereas many of the retrospective series of breast conservation patients included radiotherapy to the axilla, both dissected and undissected. In breast conservation patients, if the axilla is neither dissected nor irradiated, then the reported incidence of arm lymphedema is 0%.[7,8] If either the axilla is dissected or irradiated, but not both, then the incidence of arm lymphedema reported ranges from 2% to 27%.[7,13,20,22–31] Some of these reports also note that axillary radiotherapy either before or after axillary dissection increases this risk to between 9% and 36%.[13,20,22–28,30] The U.S. National Cancer Institute series, which included radiotherapy to the dissected axilla in some conservation patients, reported a lymphedema incidence (2 cm or greater increase in circumference) in between one-third and one-half of their patients, depending on how long they were followed.[5] Breast radiotherapy alone can increase the risk of arm edema in patients who receive axillary dissection from 4–7% without radiotherapy to 10–14% with radiotherapy.[13,20] Lymphedema developing after axillary radiotherapy without dissection appears later than that developing after combined axillary surgery and radiotherapy.[23]

Confounding observations regarding the risk of lymphedema relative to radiotherapy fields is the fact

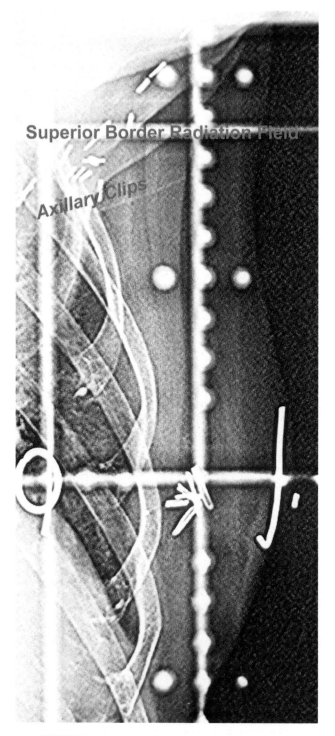

FIGURE 1. Axillary clips within the breast radiotherapy portal.

that, when giving radiotherapy to the breast through conventional portals, it is possible to incidentally radiate levels 1–2 of the axilla. Figure 1 demonstrates many of the axillary dissection clips from a level 1 and 2 dissection clearly within the superior extent of the breast radiotherapy field. In contrast, Figure 2 dem-

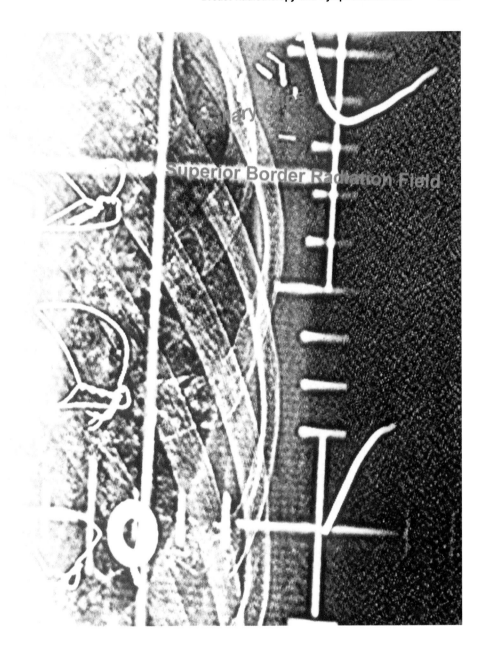

FIGURE 2. Axillary dissection clips outside of the breast radiotherapy portal.

onstrates that the clips are above the top of the breast field. Figure 3 is a typical breast radiotherapy isodose curve planned on a three-dimensional radiotherapy planning system and superimposed on an axial computed tomography image. Figure 4 is a saggital view of the same patient demonstrating that the isodose curves extend into the axilla below the humeral head and anterior to the scapula. Thus, in patients who are not radiated with formal axillary fields, it is still possible that a portion of the axilla is radiated. This may contribute to the low risk of axillary relapse in selected early stage patients treated with breast radiotherapy alone and no axillary dissection or radiotherapy.[32]

In sum, the greatest risk for arm lymphedema occurs in patients who receive both axillary surgery (great-

er than sampling) and axillary radiotherapy. Either modality alone is associated with a low risk, although this may be increased by added breast radiotherapy. Arm edema may improve with time, and one breast conservation series reported a disappearance in 38% of patients.[33] There appears to be little to no added risk engendered by radiotherapy to the supraclavicular fossa and axillary apex sparing the full axilla.[15,33–35]

Breast lymphedema

Breast lymphedema is the most frequently reported complication of breast radiotherapy.[11] Its incidence depends in large part on the extent of the reported axillary dissection, but it also may vary depending on how it is defined. It ranges from 8% to 25% in patients

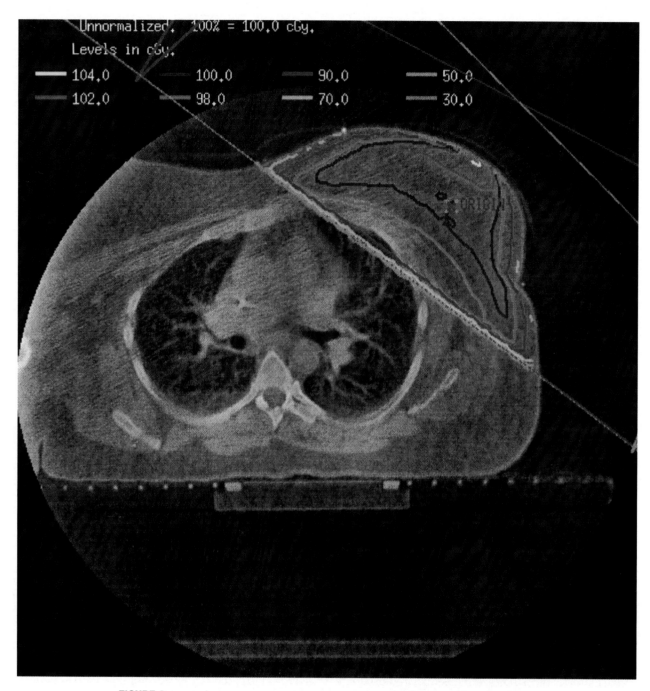

FIGURE 3. Breast radiotherapy isodose curves superimposed on an axial computed tomography section.

who receive a limited dissection and from 15% to 80% in patients who receive a full axillary dissection.[11,21] The risk of breast lymphedema in breast conservation patients undergoing axillary dissection but not receiving radiotherapy was reported in one series as 5%.[21] Chronic breast edema can be uncomfortable, can lead to repeated bouts of cellulitis, and adversely affects the cosmetic outcome of breast conservation therapy.[36] Breast edema gradually improves in most patients over a period of years,[37] although, occasionally, it can suddenly resolve.

Benefits of Breast Radiotherapy Surpass the Risk of Lymphedema

It is becoming increasingly apparent that, as the randomized clinical trials data matures, radiotherapy benefits the populations that receive it. This is true for intraductal carcinoma[38] and for invasive carcinoma,

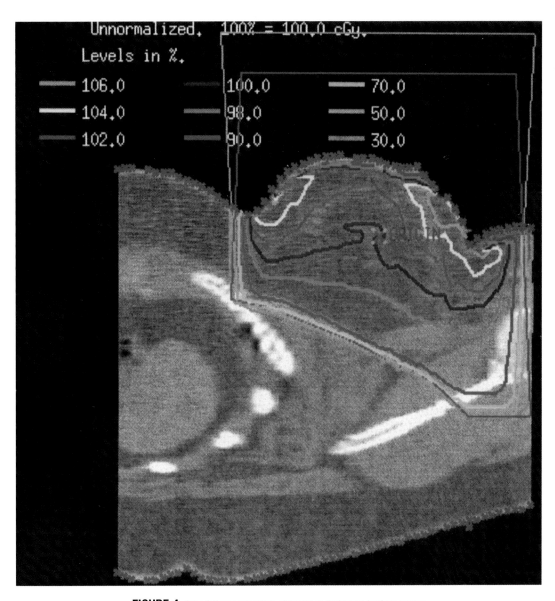

FIGURE 4. Saggital reconstruction of breast radiotherapy isodose curves.

whether it is treated by mastectomy[19,39,40] or by conservation therapy.[39,41] The benefits include substantially improved locoregional control and, in pre- and perimenopausal women who also receive chemotherapy, improved survival. Radiotherapy and chemotherapy are complementary and additive: radiotherapy enhances the survival benefit of chemotherapy, and chemotherapy enhances the locoregional control benefit of radiotherapy.

Benefits of Chest Wall and Breast Radiotherapy

The recently published trials of pre- and perimenopausal patients demonstrating improved survival with postmastectomy radiotherapy[19,40] expand the indications for radiotherapy in this population. Before those

publications, the most common indications for postmastectomy radiotherapy in the United States had been a T_3 or greater primary tumor, multiple involved axillary nodes, or an involved surgical margin.[11,42] Improved locoregional control was the outcome achieved.[39] Based on the results of these most recently reported trials, all node positive pre- and perimenopausal patients are candidates for postmastectomy radiotherapy. The radiotherapy employed included the chest wall and all three nodal stations: the internal mammary, supraclavicular, and axillary regions. Despite this extensive volume radiated, the reported incidence of arm lymphedema (in the one trial that reported it) was only 9% compared with 3% in the patients who did not receive radiotherapy.[19] How much clinical practice will actually change in the United

States is uncertain at this time. However, there is the potential of an increased prevalence of lymphedema if more patients receive postmastectomy radiotherapy.

In patients who are treated with breast conservation for invasive carcinoma, randomized trials have demonstrated that breast radiotherapy clearly results in a substantial decrease in local failure compared with breast conservation alone (an annual rate of local recurrence of ~1% with radiotherapy compared with ~4–5% without radiotherapy).[43–47] Even with very careful patient selection, breast relapse after conservation surgery alone is high (annual recurrence rate of 3.6%).[48] The outcomes reported in clinical trials with respect to locoregional control are at least as good in breast conservation patients compared with mastectomy patients.[39] The radiotherapy employed in breast conservation patients also may improve survival.[41] Also, patients are willing to accept the risks of radiotherapy to avoid a local recurrence.[49] Thus, for the foreseeable future, breast radiotherapy with its attendant risk of breast and arm edema will remain a necessary component of care for these patients.

In patients who are treated with breast conservation for intraductal carcinoma, breast radiotherapy is appropriate for the large majority of patients, substantially reducing the risk of ipsilateral breast relapse compared with breast conservation alone (annual recurrence rate of ~1.5% with radiotherapy compared with ~3.5% without radiotherapy).[38] Whether there are cohorts of patients with intraductal carcinoma who do not require breast radiotherapy is a subject of much debate.[50] Although these patients run an increased risk of breast edema after radiotherapy, the risk of arm edema should be virtually zero,[7,8,23] because they neither undergo axillary dissection nor receive formal axillary radiotherapy.

Benefits of Axillary Radiotherapy

Adequate axillary radiotherapy is comparable to adequate axillary dissection in controlling the axilla in clinical N_0 patients.[9,10,51] Because of the prognostic information afforded and the guidance regarding systemic therapy protocol provided, axillary dissection generally is preferred,[10,51] although it is controversial.[52–54] Sentinel node biopsy may replace axillary dissection in selected patients[55,56] with the potential of lower morbidity. Patients presenting with N_1 disease are managed better with surgery.[9] Axillary failure after adequate axillary dissection is so infrequent (0–2%) that routine axillary radiotherapy is not indicated.[51] However, axillary failure after inadequate axillary surgery can be quite high.[17] Axillary radiotherapy after axillary surgery with the goal of improving local control should be reserved for patients with inadequate

axillary surgery, with known gross residual disease, and possibly with N_2 disease or gross extracapsular extension,[57] although the data that justify this are scant.[9,51] Unless there is known gross residual disease, doses should be limited to 45–50 gray (Gy) in conventional fractionation, because there is no clear dose response beyond this level,[9] and there is an increased risk of complications.[26]

Whether axillary radiotherapy affords an improved survival is controversial,[9,42] with the greatest potential benefit in patients who do not receive axillary dissection.[9] The recently reported postmastectomy trials[19,40] in premenopausal women who also received chemotherapy demonstrate a survival benefit of added radiotherapy with fields that included the dissected axilla. Whether this benefit would have occurred with radiotherapy that excluded the axilla is unknown and should be investigated. Clinical judgment of the relative risks and benefits of added axillary radiotherapy will guide the practitioner until better information is available.[57]

Pathophysiology of Radiation-Related Lymphedema

Studies performed in vitro and in vivo in humans and in other mammals, have established that the lymphatic vessels are relatively insensitive to both external and endolymphatic radiation, maintaining their structural and functional integrity.[58–60] The lymphatic vessel constriction seen late postradiotherapy is thought to be due to the development of surrounding fibrous tissue. Whether radioprotectors, e.g., amifostine,[61] would be helpful in preventing this fibrosis is unknown. Although the lymphatic vessels themselves appear to be radioresistant, radiation does delay the normal growth of lymphatics into tissues repairing after surgery and inhibits the normal lymphatic proliferative response to inflammatory stimuli.[58]

In contrast, lymph nodes are radiosensitive to conventional doses of radiotherapy, responding first with lymphocyte depletion, followed by fatty replacement, and then by (usually focal) fibrosis.[62] The fibrosis is most prominent in regions of the node where preexisting tumor had been eradicated by the radiotherapy. Functionally, radiation appears to decrease the filter function of lymph nodes and to alter their immune function.[62]

This evidence suggests that early lymphedema seen after breast surgery and radiotherapy could be due to inhibition of normal lymphatic regeneration after surgical interruption and that later lymphedema could be due to delayed soft tissue fibrosis. This fibrosis can be triggered or aggravated by repeat infections that are difficult to eradicate due lymph stasis and to the impaired lymphatic proliferation response. With radiotherapy commonly now being delayed for 4–6 months after surgery in order to complete chemotherapy, perhaps less lymphedema will be seen, because the surgically disturbed tissues will have more time to heal.[63]

Patient Risk Factors for the Development of Radiation-Related Lymphedema

Patient risk factors that have been analyzed as possibly increasing the risk of lymphedema in patients receiving radiotherapy include stage at diagnosis, age, obesity, hypertension, and whether they received chemotherapy. Advanced stage at diagnosis, particularly nodal, is a well recognized risk factor for the subsequent development of lymphedema.[8,13] Complicating the assessment of how the risk of lymphedema is related to treatment is the fact that patients with more advanced nodal disease are likely to have more extensive axillary surgery along with axillary radiotherapy. These patients also are more likely to have a regional relapse of their disease.

Older age has been found in some,[7,34] but not all,[15,22] studies to be associated with an increase in the risk of lymphedema subsequent to radiotherapy. One institution found that obesity was a strong predictor of arm edema in patients who were treated with breast conservation,[33] as had been reported in mastectomy series.[15] In the authors' own experience, overweight patients with lymphedema will see improvement and, in some cases, resolution with weight loss. Hypertension was noted in one series[64] to increase the risk of arm lymphedema after axillary surgery and radiotherapy.

Chemotherapy is reported in some series[65,66] to increase the complication rate of breast radiotherapy, including arm edema, but not in others.[7,22,33,34,63] In the former series, chemotherapy was given predominantly concomitant with the radiotherapy, whereas, in the later series, it was given sequentially. In one recent series[7] reporting a significant reduction in lymphedema in breast conservation patients who received chemotherapy, the authors speculated that this was probably due to the younger age of the chemotherapy patients. However, because the chemotherapy generally was completed prior to the institution of the radiotherapy, perhaps the delay in starting radiotherapy was a salient contributor.[63]

Prevention of Radiation-Related Lymphedema

Based on the treatment- and patient-related risk factors discussed above, the following suggestions are made to reduce the incidence and prevalence of lymphedema in breast carcinoma patients who are treated with radiotherapy. These suggestions are in addition to those generally advised by surgeons after axillary dissection.[2] Increase the use of breast conservation, and, when possible, avoid posttreatment biopsies, because this increases the risk of recurrent cellulitis and breast edema.[67] Tailor the extent of axillary surgery to the risk of nodal involvement. Use axillary radiotherapy before or after axillary dissection very sparingly, if at all.[68] Only patients with the strongest indications (gross residual or N_2 disease) should be treated, and the dose to the midplane of the axilla for the treatment of microscopic residual disease should be limited to 45–50 Gy in conventional fractionation. Train patients and staff in meticulous skin care and avoidance of trauma to the arm and breast. Use antibiotics liberally whenever a cellulitis, erysipelas, or lymphangitis is suspected. Encourage overweight patients to lose weight. Consider applying stricter indications for radiotherapy in older (>55 years) patients, particularly if they are overweight. Educate the public in the value of early diagnosis, because treatment of earlier stage lesions lessens the risk of lymphedema. Support research into the use of modern radiotherapy planning systems to improve the distribution of radiation within the breast and nodal treatment fields: Support clinical trials evaluating the best use of radiotherapy in breast carcinoma, and support radiobiology research into the mechanisms of radiation-related lymphedema and its prevention.

Conclusion

Breast and arm edema continue to be risks associated with the treatment of breast carcinoma. Treatment of the axilla by both surgery and radiotherapy is rarely required, and, by avoiding both treatments, the risk of arm edema can be reduced substantially. Both surgery and radiotherapy to the breast are necessary for the large majority of patients treated by breast conservation. Thus, the risk of breast edema remains for these patients. For both arm and breast edema, the risks can be reduced by limiting the extent of breast surgery and, the extent of the axillary dissection, possibly by weight loss in the overweight patient, and by delaying radiotherapy until completion of adjuvant chemotherapy. Patient and staff education in early diagnosis, close surveillance for and prompt treatment of infections, and avoidance of trauma to the treated breast/chest wall and ipsilateral arm are important components of prevention. The risk of lymphedema is greatly surpassed by the benefits of radiotherapy in the care of the breast carcinoma patient.

REFERENCES

1. Logan V. Incidence and prevalence of lymphoedema: a literature review. *J Clin Nurs* 1995;4:213–9.

2. Petrek JA, Lerner R. Lymphedema. In: Diseases of the breast. Harris JR, Lippman ME, Morrow M, Helman S, editors. Philadelphia: Lippincott-Raven, 1996:896–900.

3. Tobin MB, Lacey HJ, Meyer L, Mortimer PS. The psychological morbidity of breast cancer—related arm swelling. *Cancer* 1993;72:3258–2.

4. Passik SD, Newman ML, Brennan M, Tunkel R. Predictors of psychological distress, sexual dysfunction and physical functioning among women with upper extremity lymphedema related to breast cancer. *Psycho-Oncol* 1995;4:255–63.

5. Gerber L, Lampert M, Wood C, Duncan M, D'Angelo T, Schain W, et al. Comparison of pain, motion, and edema after modified radical mastectomy vs. local excision with axillary dissection and radiation. *Breast Cancer Res Treat* 1992;21:132–45.

6. Brennan MJ, DePompolo RW, Garden FH. Focused review: postmastectomy lymphedema. *Arch Phys Med Rehabil* 1996; 77:74–80.

7. Kiel KD, Rademacker AW. Early-stage breast cancer: arm edema after wide excision and breast irradiation. *Radiology* 1996;198:279–83.

8. Kissin MW, Querci della Rovere G, Easton D, Westbury G. Risk of lymphoedema following the treatment of breast cancer. *Br J Surg* 1986;73:580–4.

9. Recht A, Houlihan MJ. Axillary lymph nodes and breast cancer. *Cancer* 1995;76:1491–512.

10. Falk SJ. Radiotherapy and the management of the axilla in early breast cancer. *Br J Surg* 1994;82:1277–81.

11. Perez CA, Garcia DM, Kuske RR, Levitt SH. Breast Stage T1 and T2 tumors. In: Principles and practice of radiation oncology, 2nd ed. Perez CA, Brady LW, editors. Philadelphia: JB Lippincott Company, 1992:934–6.

12. Roberts CC, Levick JR, Stanton AWB, Mortimer PS. Assessment of truncal edema following breast cancer treatment using modified Harpenden skinfold calipers. *Lymphology* 1995;28:78–88.

13. Schunemann H, Willich N. Lymphoedema of the arm after treatment of cancer of the breast. A study of 5868 cases. *Detsch Med Wschr* 1997;122:536–41.

14. Aitken DR, Minton JP. Complications associated with mastectomy. *Surg Clin North Am* 1983;63:1331–52.

15. Segerstrom K, Bjerle P, Graffman S, Nystrom A. Factors that influence the incidence of brachial oedema after treatment of breast cancer. *Scand J Plast Reconstr Hand Surg* 1992;26:223–7.

16. Bruce J. Operable cancer of the breast. A controlled clinical trial. *Cancer* 1971;28:1443–52.

17. Overgaard M, Christensen JJ, Johansen H, Nybo-Rasumssen A, Brincker H, Van Der Kooy P, et al. Postmastectomy irradiation in high-risk breast cancer patients. *Acta Oncologica* 1988;27:707–14.

18. Swedborg I, Wallgren A. The effect of a pre- and postmastectomy radiotherapy on the degree of edema, shoulder-joint mobility, and gripping force. *Cancer* 1981;47:877–81.

19. Ragaz J, Jackson SM, Le N, Plenderleith I, Spinelli J, Basco VE, et al. Adjuvant radiotherapy and chemotherapy in node-positive premenopausal women with breast cancer. *N Engl J Med* 1997;337:956–62.

20. Moffat FL, Senofsky GM, David K, Clark KC, Robinson DS, Ketcham AS, et al. Axillary node dissection for early breast cancer: some is good, but all is better. *J Surg Oncol* 1992;51:8–13.

21. Senofsky GM, Moffat FL, Davis K, Masri MM, Clark KC, Robinson DS, et al. Total axillary lymphadenectomy in the management of breast cancer. *Arch Surg* 1991;126:1336–42.

22. Larson D, Weinstein M, Goldberg I, Silver B, Recht A, Cady B, et al. Edema of the arm as a function of the extent of axillary surgery in patients with Stage I–II carcinoma of breast treated with primary radiotherapy. *Int J Radiat Oncol Biol Phys* 1986;12:1575–82.

23. Pierquin B, Mazeron J, Glaubiger D. Conservative treatment of breast cancer in Europe: report of the Groupe Europeen de Curietherapie. *Radiother Oncol* 1986;6:187–98.

24. Cabanes PA, Salmon RJ, Vilcoq JR, Durand JC, Fourquet A, Gautier C, et al. Value of axillary dissection in addition to lumpectomy and radiotherapy in early breast cancer. *Lancet* 1992;339:1245–8.

25. Pierquin B, Huart J, Raynal M, Otmezguine Y, Calitchi E, Mazeron J, et al. Conservative treatment for breast cancer: long-term results (15 years). *Radiother Oncol* 1991;20:16–23.

26. Delouch G, Bachelot F, Premont M, Kurtz JM. Conservation treatment of early breast cancer: long term results and complications. *Int J Radiat Oncol Biol Phys* 1987;13:29–34.

27. Touboul E, Buffat L, Lefranc JP, Blondon J, Deniaud E, Mammar H, et al. Possibility of conservative local treatment after combined chemotherapy and preoperative irradiation for locally advanced noninflammatory breast cancer. *Int J Radiat Oncol Biol Phys* 1996;1534:1019–28.

28. Siegel BM, Mayzel K, Love SM. Level I and II axillary dissection in the treatment of early-stage breast cancer. An analysis of 259 consecutive patients. *Arch Surg* 1990;125:1144–7.

29. Kantorowitz DA, Poulter CA, Rubin P, Patterson E, Sobel SH, Sischy B, et al. Treatment of breast cancer with segmental mastectomy alone or segmental mastectomy plus radiation. *Radiat Oncol* 1989;15:141–50.

30. Dewar JA, Sarrazin D, Benhamou E, Petit JY, Benhamou S, Arriagada R, et al. Management of the axilla in conservatively treated breast cancer: 592 patients treated at Institut Gustave-Roussy. *Int J Radiat Oncol Biol Phys* 1987;13:475–81.

31. Osborne MP, Ormiston N, Harmer CL, McKinna JA, Baker J, Greening WP. Breast conservation in the treatment of early breast cancer. A 20-year follow-up. *Cancer* 1984;53:349–55.

32. Wong JS, Recht A, Beard CJ, Busse PM, Cady B, Chaffey JT, et al. Treatment outcome after tangential radiation therapy without axillary dissection in patients with early-stage breast cancer and clinically negative axillary nodes. *Int J Radiat Gncol Biol Phys* 1997;39:915–20.

33. Werner RS, McCormick B, Petrek J, Cox L, Cirrincione C, Gray J, et al. Arm edema in conservatively managed breast cancer: obesity is a major predictive factor. *Radiology* 1991; 180:177–84.

34. Pezner RP, Patterson MP, Hill LR, Lipsett JA, Desai KR, Vora N, et al. Arm lymphedema in patients treated conservatively for breast cancer: relationship to patient age and axillary node dissection technique. *Int J Radiat Oncol Biol Phys* 1986;12:2079–83.

35. Danoff BF, Pajak TF, Solin LJ, Goodman RL. Excisional biopsy, axillary node dissection and definitive radiotherapy for Stages I and II breast cancer. *Int J Radiat Oncol Biol Phys* 1985;11:479–83.

36. McCormick B, Yahalom J, Cox L, Shank B, Massie MJ. The patient's perception of her breast following radiation and limited surgery. *Int J Radiat Oncol Biol Phys* 1989;17:1299–302.

37. Clarke D, Martinez A, Cox RS, Goffinet DR. Breast edema following staging axillary node dissection in patients with breast carcinoma treated by radical radiotherapy. *Cancer* 1982;49:2295–9.

38. Fisher B, Dignam J, Wolmark N, Mamounas E, Costantino J, Poller W, et al. Lumpectomy and radiation therapy for the treatment of intraductal breast cancer: findings from national surgical adjuvant breast and bowel project B-17. *J Clin Oncol* 1998;16:441–52.

39. Early Breast Cancer Trialists' Collaborative Group. Effects of radiotherapy and surgery in early breast cancer. An overview of the randomized trials. *New Engl J Med* 1995;333:1444–1455.

40. Overgaard M, Hansen PS, Overgaard J, Rose C, Andersson M, Bach, et al. Postoperative radiotherapy in high-risk premenopausal women with breast cancer who receive adjuvant chemotherapy. *N Engl J Med* 1997;337:949–1147.

41. Morris A, Morris RD, Wilson JF, White J, Steinberg S, Okunieff P, et al. Breast-conserving in early-stage breast cancer: a meta-analysis of 10-year survival. *Cancer J* 1997;3:6–11.

42. Levitt SH. Controversies in the management of the lymphatics in breast cancer. *Front Radiat Ther Oncol* 1994;28:79–91.

43. Fisher B, Redmond C. Lumpectomy for breast cancer. An update of the NSABP experience. *Monogr J Natl Cancer Inst* 1992;11:7–13.

44. Veronesi U, Luini A, Del Vecchio M, Greco M, Galimberti V, Merson M, et al. Radiotherapy after breast preserving surgery in women with localized cancer of the breast. *N Engl J Med* 1993;328:1587–91.

45. Clark RM, McColloch PB, Levine MN, Lipa M, Wilkinson RH, Mahoney LJ, et al. Randomized clinical trial to assess the effectiveness of breast irradiation following lumpectomy and axillary dissection for node-negative breast cancer. *J Natl Cancer Inst* 1992;84:683–9.

46. The Uppsala-Orebro Breast Cancer Study Group. Sector resection with or without postoperative radiotherapy for Stage I breast cancer: A randomized trial. *J Natl Cancer Inst* 1990;82:277–82.

47. Liljegren G, Holmberg L, Adami H-O, Westman G, Graffman S, Bergh J. Sector resection with or without postoperative radiotherapy for Stage I breast cancer: five-year results of a randomized trial. *J Natl Cancer Inst* 1994;86:717–22.

48. Schnitt SJ, Hayman J, Gelman R, Eberlein TJ, Love SM, Mayzel K, et al. A prospective study of conservative surgery alone in the treatment of selected patients with Stage I breast cancer. *Cancer* 1996;77:1094–100.

49. Hayman JA, Fairclough DL, Harris JR, Weeks JC. Patient preferences concerning the trade-off between the risks and benefits of routine radiation therapy after conservative surgery for early-stage breast cancer. *J Clin Oncol* 1997;15:1252–60.

50. Silverstein MJ, Lagios MD. Use of predictors of recurrence to plan therapy for DCIS of the breast. *Oncology* 1997;2:393–415.

51. Recht A, Pierce S, Abner A, Vicini F, Osteen RT, Love SM, et al. Regional nodal failure after conservative surgery and radiotherapy for early-stage breast carcinoma. *J Clin Oncol* 1991;9:988–96.

52. Lin PP, Allison DC, Wainstock J, Miller KD, Dooley WC, Friedman N, et al. Impact of axillary lymph node dissection on the therapy of breast cancer patients. *J Clin Oncol* 1993;11:1536–44.

53. Cady B. Is axillary lymph node dissection necessary in routine management of breast cancer? No 17. In: Important advances in oncology. DeVita VT, Hellman S, Rosenberg S, editors. Philadelphia: Lippincott-Raven, 1996:251–65.

54. Moore MP, Kinne DW. Is axillary lymph node dissection necessary in the routine management of breast cancer? Yes 16. In: Important advances in oncology. DeVita VT, Hellman S, Rosenberg S, editors. Philadelphia: Lippincott-Raven, 1996:245–50.

55. Greco M, Agresti R, Raselli R, Giovannazzi R, Veronesi U. Axillary dissection can be avoided in selected breast cancer patients: analysis of 401 cases. *Anticancer Res* 1996;16:3913–7.

56. Veronesi U, Paganelli G, Galimberti V, Viale G, Zurrida S, Dedoni M, et al. Sentinel-node biopsy to avoid axillary dissection in breast cancer with negative lymph nodes. *Lancet* 1997;349:1864–7.

57. Lichter AS, Fraass BA, Yanke B. Treatment techniques in the conservative management of breast cancer. *Semin Radiat Oncol* 1992;2:94–106.

58. Van Den Brenk HAS. The effect of ionizing radiations on the regeneration and behavior of mammalian lymphatics. In vivo studies in Sandison Clark chambers. *Am J Roentgenol Radiat Therapy Nucl Med* 1957;78:837–49.

59. Ariel IM, Resnick MI, Oropeza R. The effects of irradiation (external and internal) on lymphatic dynamics. *Am J Roentgenol Radiat Ther Nucl Med* 1967;99:404–14.

60. Lenzi M, Bassani G. The effect of radiation on the lymph and on the lymph vessels. *Radiology* 1963;80:814–7.

61. Tannehill SP, Mehta MP. Amifostine and radiation therapy: past, present and future. *Semin Oncol* 1996;23:69–77.

62. Fajardo LF. Effects of ionizing radiation on lymph nodes. *Front Radiat Ther Oncol* 1994;28:37–45.

63. Keramoupoulos A, Txionou C, Minaretzis D, Michalas S, Anavantinos D. Arm morbidity following treatment of breast cancer with total axillary dissection: a multivariated approach. *Oncology* 1993;50:445–9.

64. Bohler FK, Rhomberg W, Doringer W. Hypertonie als Riskofactor fur erohte Nebenwirkunsraten im Rahmen der Mammakarzinombestrahlung. *Strahlenther Onkol* 1992;168:344–9.

65. Danoff BF, Goodman RL, Glick JH, Hallen DG, Pajak TF. The effects of adjuvant chemotherapy on cosmesis and complications in patients with breast cancer treated by definitive irradiation. *Int J Radiat Oncol Biol Phys* 1983;9:1625–30.

66. Ray GR, Fish VJ, Marmor JB, Rogoway W, Kushlan P, Arnold C, et al. Impact of adjuvant chemotherapy on cosmesis and complications in Stages I and II carcinoma of the breast treated by biopsy and radiation therapy. *Int J Radiat Oncol Biol Phys* 1984;10:837–41.

67. Pezner RD, Lorant JA, Terz J, Ben-Ezra J, Odom-Maryon T, Luk KH. Wound-healing complications following biopsy of the irradiated breast. *Arch Surg* 1992;127:321–5.

68. Kirshbaum M. The development, implementation and evaluation of guidelines for the management of breast cancer related lymphoedema. *Eur J Cancer Care (Engl)* 1996;5:246–51.

American Cancer Society Lymphedema Workshop

Supplement to **Cancer**

The Pathophysiology of Lymphedema

Peter S. Mortimer, M.D.

Department of Physiological Medicine (Dermatology), St. George's Hospital Medical School, London, United Kingdom.

BACKGROUND. All edemas result from an imbalance between capillary filtration and tissue (lymph) drainage. This basic approach was adopted to investigate mechanisms for chronic arm edema following breast carcinoma treatment.

METHODS. A review of causes of lymphedema is presented plus the traditional pathophysiology of breast carcinoma related lymphedema (postmastectomy edema; PME). A summary of recent research that explored capillary filtration as a surrogate for lymph flow in the steady state is presented.

RESULTS. A reduced interstitial protein concentration (relative to plasma) argues against lymphatic obstruction. Evidence exists that total arm blood flow (in some patients) and vascular bed size are increased in PME.

CONCLUSIONS. The primary insult to the axillary lymphatic system by surgery and radiotherapy presumably is the root cause of PME; however, there is strong evidence to suggest that hemodynamic factors are contributory to the chronic swelling. *Cancer* 1998;83:2798–802. © *1998 American Cancer Society.*

KEYWORDS: lymphedema, breast carcinoma, microcirculation, edema.

Presented at the American Cancer Society Lymphedema Workshop, New York, New York, February 20–22, 1998.

Supported by the Wellcome Trust, the Frances and Augustus Newman Foundation, and the Charles Skey Charitable Trust.

The author thanks Dr. A. Stanton, Ph.D., Principal Investigator, and Prof. J.R. Levick, D.Sc., Co-Supervisor.

Dr. Mortimer is a Consultant Skin Physician to St. George's and Royal Marsden Hospitals, London, and a Reader in Dermatology, University of London.

Address for reprints: Peter S. Mortimer, M.D., Department of Physiological Medicine (Dermatology), St. George's Hospital Medical School, Cranmer Terrace, London SW17 0RE, United Kingdom.

Received July 2, 1998; accepted August 20, 1998.

Edema represents an increase in interstitial fluid volume sufficient to manifest with swelling. Any edema, whatever the underlying cause, is due to an imbalance between capillary filtration and lymph drainage.[1] Most examples of limb edema are caused by an increase in capillary filtration, overwhelming lymph drainage capacity (e.g., heart failure, nephrotic syndrome). Lymphedema strictly occurs when swelling is due to a failure of lymph drainage in circumstances in which capillary filtration is not increased. Because of the dynamic and ever-changing balance between capillary filtration and lymph drainage, few clinical edemas are likely to be purely a "filtration edema" or "lymphedema." In this article, the possible mechanisms leading to lymphedema are discussed with particular reference to breast carcinoma-related lymphedema (postmastectomy edema; PME).

The Physiology of Lymph Drainage

The lymph system is a one-way drainage route designed to rid the "tissues" of unwanted material and excess fluid. It therefore represents a garbage route and overflow pipe, with its essential function being to return to the blood vascular compartment protein, colloids, and particulate matter too large to reenter the blood compartment directly.[2]

Two types of lymphatic vessel exist: first, the smaller initial lymphatic, which includes the smallest lymphatic capillary and the larger precollector vessel,[3] and, second, the collecting lymphatic vessel into which the precollectors drain. The collecting lymphatics are the main limb lymphatic vessels that provide the afferent flow to the lymph nodes. They behave like a series of smooth muscle hearts that are responsible mainly for the propulsion of lymph centripetally.[4] Intrin-

TABLE 1
Lymph Drainage Failure

| Reduced lymph-conducting pathways | Mechanism | | |
	Hypertrophy or hyperplasia of lymphatic vessels	Functional failure	Obstructed lymphatics
Possible causes			
	Lymphangiomatosis, lymphatic malformations	Valvular failure	Lymph node abnormalities (e.g., fibrosis)
Aplasia or hypoplasia of whole vessel			"Scarring" from lymphadenectomy,
Acquired obliteration of lymphatic lumen (e.g., lymphangiothrombosis, lymphangitis)	Megalymphatics	Disordered contractility	radiotherapy, or infection

sic pumping of collecting vessels is the essential motor for lymph propulsion, but flow can be only as good as the supply of lymph to these collectors. In other words, the physiology is identical to Starling's law of the heart.

The supply of lymph from the initial lymphatics is dependent on a different mechanism. Flow of interstitial fluid and macromolecules into and consequently along initial lymphatics is caused by intermittent changes in hydrostatic and oncotic pressures locally[5] (convective flow). Deformation or movement of the tissues by surface pressure or underlying muscle contractions and by other contractile structures, such as arterioles, causes expansion or compression of the initial lymphatics. The compression phase forces lymph along initial lymphatics. Valves in both initial and collecting lymphatics ensure that flow is unidirectional. Knowledge of normal lymphatic physiology is clearly important for understanding reasons for its failure in lymphedema.

Causes of Lymph Drainage Failure

Lymphedema arises when an intrinsic fault develops within the lymph-conducting pathways (primary lymphedema) or when damage occurs from one or more factors originating outside the lymphatic system, such as surgical removal of lymph nodes (secondary lymphedema; Table 1). In truth, the term secondary lymphedema is used when a cause can be identified, and primary lymphedema is used when a cause cannot be identified.

Although the exact pathogenesis of lymphedema often is unclear, it is more than likely that the lymph pump fails. In the commonest form of primary lymphedema, insufficient numbers of lymphatic collectors, as demonstrated by lymphographic studies, are observed.[6] However, a mystery remains whether the collecting vessels are abnormal at birth. In the majority of cases in which "distal hypoplasia" occurs, lymphedema develops later in life either at or after puberty (lymphedema praecox) or sometimes much

later in life (lymphedema tarda), yet the abnormality is considered congenital. It is possible that the defect may be programmed from birth (as suggested by the familial nature of such cases of primary lymphedema) and that an atrophy or early aging process develops to cause lymph drainage failure. The recent demonstration of severe atrophy of the smooth muscle layer in proximal limb lymphatics with relative sparing of distal vessels suggests that a degenerative process may begin proximally and spread distally.[7] This could help explain the variable time for onset of lymphedema in both primary and secondary forms.

Milroy's disease is a rare and specific form of primary lymphedema that is inherited and in which the onset is either at or soon after birth, yet the term frequently is used interchangeably with primary lymphedema. Unlike other forms of primary lymphedema, initial lymphatics appear absent.[8]

At the other end of the spectrum from hypoplasia/aplasia, lymph vessels may be hyperplastic. Lymphatics that are excessive in number and size at times may be considered a tumor or at least a form of hamartomatous malformation (lymphangioma). Lymphatic collectors that are enlarged and dilated are referred to as megalymphatics. Lymph reflux seems commonplace with such vessel abnormalities due to valvular insufficiency.[9]

Valvular failure may arise for reasons other than congenitally determined lymphatic abnormalities. Mechanical obstruction like what occurs following surgical procedures, results in outflow resistance and a rise in lymphatic pressure. The resulting lymphatic dilation is likely to cause valve incompetence and hence, explains the backflow of lymph, particularly toward the skin ("dermal backflow").[9] Although most acquired forms of lymphedema in developed countries result from carcinoma therapy (surgery and/or radiotherapy) various forms of infection also can undermine lymph drainage. It is assumed that filariasis results from mechanical obstruction by the worms, but products of the filarial parasites have been shown to depress lymphatic contractility.[10] Recurrent lymphangitis/cellulitis can lead to gradual obliteration of lymphatic vessels, and it is possible that lymphangiothrombosis may do the same.

One of the difficulties in elucidating the cause of any lymphedema is a paucity of sensitive investigatory methods. No means exist for exploring lymphatic contractility in humans, and methods for imaging lymph vessels in vivo are limited.

Breast Carcinoma-Related Lymphedema (PME)

Chronic edema of the arm, commonly called lymphedema or postmastectomy edema (PME), was described first as a side effect of mastectomy operations by Halstead in 1921.[11] Although there has been a trend toward more conservative surgery and greater use of radiotherapy, PME remains a common iatrogenic problem, with a cumulative incidence of 28% in a large cohort of breast carcinoma patients studied in the south of England.[12]

Natural History

Breast carcinoma rarely presents with arm swelling, even when the axillary nodes are infiltrated with tumor. Relapsed carcinoma, however, can cause PME and always must be considered in any patient presenting with arm swelling who is considered to be in remission following initial carcinoma treatment.

Following surgery, i.e., various degrees of axillary dissection, arm edema may develop immediately and either settle or persist. Alternatively, swelling may develop months or years after the original uneventful carcinoma treatment. After an initial rapid expansion, arm volume tends to stabilize and remains in a relatively steady state.

The swollen arm, which can be as much as twice the normal size, is disfiguring and commonly causes functional impairment, a feeling of heaviness and aching, psychosocial maladjustment and psychological morbidity.[13] There is no consistency in the site of the swelling, which may affect part or all of the limb, nor in the quality of the swelling, which may be brawny, or "fatty," or sometimes easily pitting. Like other forms of lymphedema, recurrent acute inflammatory episodes ("cellulitis" or "erysipelas") can affect up to one-third of patients. Such attacks increase swelling and compound the problem. Although the cause of PME is undoubtedly the breast carcinoma treatment, the underlying pathophysiologic mechanisms involved in the swelling seem less clear cut in light of recent research.

Traditional View of Pathophysiology

The pathogenesis at first seems self evident, namely, that damage to the axillary lymphatic system caused by surgery and/or radiotherapy impairs lymph drainage from the arm. Lymphangiography during the latent phase (posttreatment but before swelling) shows dilation of the main collecting lymphatics in the arm.[14] Contrast medium appears to be held up at the operation site in the axilla. Normally, lymph from the superficial system (superficial to the fascia) drains into the deep lymphatic system across fascial connections, and these connections can be visualized. Once edema has developed, the deep lymphatic system is no longer visualized and there is much dermal collateralisation and retrograde flow from deep vessels to the superficial skin lymphatics (dermal backflow).[15] This indicates valvular incompetence.

In general, far more tissue damage is necessary to produce experimental lymphedema than is ever created from breast carcinoma treatments. This suggests that factors in addition to lymphatic obstruction are needed to generate PME.

Protein Concentration in PME

Swelling, once it is established, reaches a steady state. If lymph drainage is reduced, then so is capillary filtration, and, consequently, protein concentration (and interstitial osmotic pressure) should rise. Recent work analyzing interstitial fluid extracted by using the Wick technique from both swollen and nonswollen arms demonstrated that, contrary to expectations, protein concentrations were lower in the swollen arm. Indeed, protein concentration correlated negatively with the severity of arm swelling[16] (Fig. 1). The most likely explanation for these findings was that there was a vascular contribution to the swelling, and increased capillary filtration seemed possible.

Blood Vascular Factors in PME

The contribution of venous obstruction to the development of swelling has long been controversial. Altered venous anatomy by venography has suggested obstruction,[17] more recently, investigation of venous outflow using duplex Doppler ultrasound revealed that only 30% of patients were normal.[18] However, measurement of venous pressures in PME arms has not demonstrated any consistent increase.[19]

Other possible vascular mechanisms that would raise the net filtration rate and so increase the fluid load on a weakened lymphatic system include 1) failure to maintain precapillary resistance (allowing blood flow and capillary pressure to rise) and 2) an increase in blood vessel numbers (angiogenesis), lead-

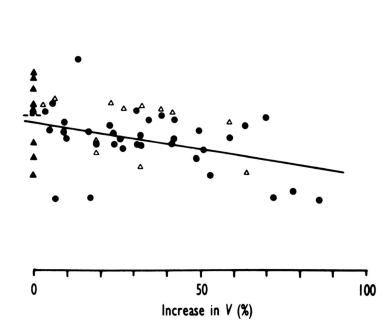

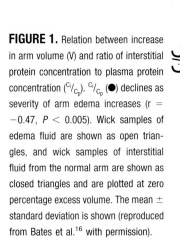

FIGURE 1. Relation between increase in arm volume (V) and ratio of interstitial protein concentration to plasma protein concentration (c_i/c_p). c_i/c_p (●) declines as severity of arm edema increases ($r = -0.47$, $P < 0.005$). Wick samples of edema fluid are shown as open triangles, and wick samples of interstitial fluid from the normal arm are shown as closed triangles and are plotted at zero percentage excess volume. The mean ± standard deviation is shown (reproduced from Bates et al.[16] with permission).

ing to an increased surface area for filtration. Evidence for hemodynamic changes had been reported previously.[20] Mean axillosubclavian blood flow measured by spectral Doppler demonstrated a 68% increase on the swollen side.[21] Furthermore, by using venous occlusion plethysmography, total arm blood flow (volume × blood flow/mL) was increased in the majority of patients but not blood flow per unit volume of arm.[22] The finding of increased blood flow to the whole arm raises two possibilities: 1) vasodilatation of existing resistance vessels and 2) formation of new vessels in parallel to existing ones.

Regarding the first possibility, sympathetic vasoconstrictor control and sympathetic vasodilator control were found to be normal in the PME arm, but local vasodilator control (postischaemic hyperaemia) was impaired.[23] No evidence for sustained vasodilatation and, hence, for a rise in capillary pressure was found. Regarding the second possibility, a preliminary study of blood capillary density has found an increase in skin on the swollen side, suggesting an increase in total capillary numbers in the PME arm.[24] Capillary angiogenesis could be increasing the surface area for an exchange and so increase the filtration load.

CONCLUSION

The primary insult to the axillary lymphatic system by surgery and radiotherapy is presumably the root cause of PME, but there is strong evidence to suggest that hemodynamic factors contribute to sustaining edema even if they are not causal. The basic rule that all edemas result from an imbalance between capillary

filtration and tissue (lymph) drainage, in itself, demands consideration of the state of the microcirculation as well as of the lymphatic drainage. Total arm blood flow and vascular bed size appear to be increased in PME, factors that will increase capillary filtration in the limb overall. One of the problems in studying PME is that patients are investigated at one moment in time during an evolving process. The pathophysiology of PME is not simply lymphatic obstruction, and unravelling the complex sequence of events in PME will need research not only on established PME but also at its earlier, latent stage.

REFERENCES

1. Levick JR. An introduction to cardiovascular physiology, 2nd ed. Oxford: Butterworth-Heinemann, 1995.
2. Yoffey JM, Courtice JM. Lymphatics, lymph and the lymphomyeloid complex. New York: Academic Press, 1970.
3. Kubik S, Manestar M. Anatomy of the lymph capillaries and pre-collectors of the skin. In: The initial lymphatics. Bollinger A, Partsch H, Wolfe JN, editors. Stuttgart: Georg Thieme Verlag, 1985:66–74.
4. Smith RO. Lymphatic contractility: a possible mechanism of lymphatic vessels for the transport of lymph. *J Exp Med* 1949;90:497–509.
5. Roddie IC. Lymph transport mechanisms in peripheral lymphatics. *New Physiol Sci* 1990;5:85–9.
6. Browse NL, Stewart G. Lymphedema: pathophysiology and classification. *J Cardiovasc Surg* 1985;6:91–106.
7. Koshima I, Kawada S, Moriguchi J, Kajiwara Y. Ultrastructural observations of lymphatic vessels in lymphedema in human extremities. *Plast Reconstr Surg* 1996;97:397–407.
8. Bollinger A, Isenring G, Franzeck UK, Brunner U. Aplasia of superficial lymphatic capillaries in hereditary and connatal lymphedema (Milroy's disease). *Lymphology* 1983;16:27–30.

9. Kinmonth JB. Lymphatics, lymphology and diseases of the chyle and lymph systems. 2nd ed. London: Edward Arnold, 1982.

10. Kaiser L, Mupanumunda M, Williams JF, Brugia Pahangi-induced contractility of bovine mesenteric lymphatics studied in vitro: a role for filarial factors in the development of lymphedema. *Am J Trop Med Hyg* 1996;54:386–90.

11. Halstead WS. The swelling of the arm after operations for cancer of the breast-elephantiasis chirurgica—its cause and prevention. *Bull John Hopkins Hosp* 1921;32:309–13.

12. Mortimer PS, Bates SO, Brassington HD, Stanton AWB, Strachan DP, Levick JR. The prevalence of arm edema following treatment for breast cancer. *Q J Med* 1996;89:377–80.

13. Tobin MB, Lacey HJ, Meyer L, Mortimer PS. The psychological morbidity of breast cancer related arm swelling. *Cancer* 1993;72:3248–52.

14. Hughes JH, Patel AR. Swelling of the arm following radical mastectomy. *Br J Surg* 1966;53:4–15.

15. Feldman MG, Kohan P, Edelman S, Jacobson JH. Lymphangiographic studies in obstructive lymphedema of the upper extremity. *Surgery* 1966;59:935–43.

16. Bates DO, Levick JR, Mortimer PS. Changes in macromolecular compositions of interstitial fluid from swollen arms after breast cancer treatment and its implications. *Clin Sci* 1993;85:737–46.

17. Veal JR. The pathological basis for swelling of the arm following radical amputation of the breast. *Surg Gynecol Obstet* 1938;67:752–60.

18. Svensson WE, Mortimer PS, Tohno E, Cosgrove DO. Colour Doppler demonstrates venous flow abnormalities in breast cancer patients with chronic arm swelling. *Eur J Cancer* 1994;30A:657–60.

19. Bates DO, Levick JR, Mortimer PS. Subcutaneous interstitial fluid pressure and arm volume in lymphedema. *Int J Microcirc* 1992;11:359–73.

20. Jacobsson S. Studies of the blood circulation in lymphedematous limbs. *Scand J Plast Reconstr Surg* 1967;3(Suppl):4–81.

21. Svensson WE, Mortimer PS, Tohno E, Cosgrove DO. Increased arterial inflow demonstrated by Doppler ultrasound in arm swelling following breast cancer treatment. *Eur J Cancer* 1994;30A:661–4.

22. Stanton AWB, Holroyd B, Northfield JW, Levick JR, Mortimer PS. Forearm blood flow measured by venous occlusion plethysmography in healthy subjects and in women with postmastectomy oedema. *Vasc Med* 1998;3:3–8.

23. Stanton AWB, Levick JR, Mortimer PS. Assessment of cutaneous vascular control in the arms of women with postmastectomy edema. *Exp Physiol* 1996;81:447–64.

24. Roberts CC, Stanton AWB, Pullen J, Bull RH, Levick JR, Mortimer PS. Skin microvascular architecture and perfusion studied in human postmastectomy edema by intravital video-capillaroscopy. *Int J Microcirc* 1994;14:327–34.

American Cancer Society Lymphedema Workshop

Supplement to **Cancer**

A Review of Measures of Lymphedema

Lynn H. Gerber, M.D.

Warren G. Magnuson Clinical Center, National Institutes of Health, Bethesda, Maryland.

BACKGROUND. Lymphedema usually is identified by patients, and rarely is it screened for routinely. Many assessments have been reported and have been used in evaluating a variety of treatments for lymphedema.

METHODS. A review of the literature was undertaken.

RESULTS. Five frequently used measures of lymphedema include circumferential measures of limbs at various points (usually at bony landmarks); volumetric measures using limb submersion in water; skin tonometry, in which soft tissue compression is quantified; imaging techniques to describe tissue characteristics as well as to quantify soft tissue swelling (magnetic resonance imaging and computerized tomography; and ultrasound with and without Doppler flow studies for volumetric measures. Circumferential measures with calculations designed to compute limb volumes and volumetric measures are used most frequently, but these have some difficulty with reliability. No significant effort has been made to develop a patient based questionnaire that describes the size as well as the impact of lymphedema on an individual's functional level.

CONCLUSIONS. Existing physical measures of lymphedema are available that are easy to use, inexpensive, have limited reliability, and do not address the issue of functional impact. Imaging techniques may provide valuable qualitative and quantitative information in selected populations. *Cancer* **1998;83:2803–4.**
© *1998 American Cancer Society.*

KEYWORDS: lymphedema, assessment, circumferential measurements, volumetrics, tonometry, ultrasound.

Presented at the American Cancer Society Lymphedema Workshop, New York, New York, February 20–22, 1998.

Address for reprints: Lynn H. Gerber, M.D., Warren G. Magnuson Clinical Center, National Institutes of Health, Bethesda, MD 20892.

Received July 2, 1998; accepted August 20, 1998.

The woman who had undergone treatment for breast carcinoma is subject to adverse as well as curative effects of surgical, radiation, and chemo-/biologic therapeutics. Lymphedema of the chest wall of the breast for those who undergo breast sparing procedures and for each segment of the upper extremity (arm, forearm, and hand) has been reported.[1] Knowledge about the incidence, severity, and rate at which it resolves when treated is lacking. This in part is because measurement techniques have not been applied widely. There is an as yet, unmet need for easy, low risk, cost effective, and accurate measures of lymphedema that can be used routinely at bedside and clinic. Developing good measures will help in determining the incidence of the problem, its response to treatments, and the impact of lymphedema on function.[2]

Typically, it is patients who observe a change in status. They note inability to wear rings, bracelets, and watches, or they have difficulty fitting into clothing. Commonly, they will observe a change in the appearance of their skin: It appears tight or shiny, has fewer folds, and feels stiff or taut. Occasionally, there is limited range of motion of elbow, wrist, or fingers.

The health care provider often observes pitting with digital compression, loss of skin folds, or asymmetry of the extremities.

The use of circumferential measurements in quantifying lymphedema has been the most frequently used method.[3–5] Techniques have included measuring the circumference of bony landmarks, (ulnar styloid, olecranon, metacarpal phalangeal joints) or measuring equilinear segments of the arm and computing volume, (i.e., 100 mm length, measuring the circumference at the proximal and distal border, and calculating the volume [volume = π (circumference/$2\pi)^2$h].

Problems with measurements are many. Using bony landmarks defines segments that are not equidistant. Measuring the circumference of the hand is an inaccurate way of determining volume because of its highly irregular shape.

Another method of measuring volume is by water displacement. The limb is submerged in a cylinder filled to a known level of water. The amount of water displaced by the submerged limbs is equivalent to its volume.[6]

The third frequently used method is that of a tissue tonometer.[7] This measures the amount of pressure necessary to depress the skin a specified amount. This degree of compressibility has been correlated with circumference and, thus, with the amount of lymphedema.[8]

The reliability of these techniques has been tested and, to some extent, compared with one another.[7] Nonetheless, circumferential measures have been the most frequently used technique, probably because of the ease with which they can be applied, the low cost, and the ability to generate quantitative data.

Quantitative measures of soft tissue edema also can be assessed by using magnetic resonance imaging (MRI), computerized tomography (CT), and ultrasound. These measures have been used to describe the characteristics of tissue involvement as well.[9–11]

Recently, reports have been published that describe the problem of lymph stasis in which an attempt to image flow through the lymphatic system has been made. Much of this work has been done in patients with filariasis or in those who are evaluated pre- and postlymphatic-venous-lymphatic anastomoses. Imaging techniques with isotopic scintigraphy and Doppler venous flow metrics have been combined to evaluate treatment.[12]

Many techniques are available for lymphedema assessment. What is needed is to encourage the use of measurements on a more routine base. This type of measurement should be easy to use, accessible, inexpensive, reliable, and quantifiable. For those studies in which outcome measures need to be highly sensitive, quantitative imaging techniques probably are more sensitive but also are less accessible and more expensive.

A fruitful area for research and development is to devise a patient-administered questionnaire to assess the degree of swelling and its impact on function. It would not be difficult to ask patients to evaluate quantitatively the amount of skin change, pitting, increase in size, stiffness, and the impact these changes have on daily routines, work, and recreational activity. This would give use valuable incidence information as well as an understanding of the input lymphedema has on the daily activities and life of the breast carcinoma patient.

REFERENCES

1. Kissin MW, Querci Della Rovere G, Easton D, et al. The risk of lymphedema following the treatment of breast cancer. *Br J Surg* 1986;73:580–4.
2. Sitzia J, Stanton AW, Badger C. A review of outcome indicators in the treatment of chronic limb edema. *Clin Rehabil* 1997;11:181–91.
3. Foldi E, Foldi M, Clodius L. The lymphedema chaos: a lancet. *Ann Plast Surg* 1989;22:505–15.
4. Bunce IH, Mirolo BR, Hennessy JM, et al. Post mastectomy lymphoedema treatment and measurement. *Med J Aust* 1994;161:125–8.
5. Mortimer PS. Investigation and management of lymphoedema. *Vasc Med Rev* 1990;1:1–20.
6. Kaulesar Sukal DMKS, den Hoed PT, Johannes EJ, et al. Direct and indirect methods for the quantification of leg volume: comparison between water displacement volumetry, the dish model method and the frustum sign model method, using the correlation coefficient and the limits of agreement. *J Biomed Eng* 1993;15:477–80.
7. Clodius L, Deak L, Piller NB. A new instrument for the evaluation of tissue tonicity in lymphoedema. *Lymphology* 1976;9:1–5.
8. Piller NB, Clodius L. The use of a tissue tonometer as a diagnostic aid in extremity lymphoedema: a determination of its conservative treatment with benzo-pyrones. *Lymphology* 1976;9:127–32.
9. Duwell S, Hagspiel KD, Zuber J, et al. Swollen lower extremity: role of MR imaging. *Radiology* 1992;184:227–31.
10. Stewart G, Hurst PAG, Lea Thomas M, et al. CAT scanning in the management of the lymphoedematous limb. *Immunol Haematol Res* 1983;2:241–3.
11. Flippetti M, Santoro E, Graziano F, et al. Modern therapeutic approaches to post mastectomy brachial lymphedema. *Microsurgery* 1994;15:604–10.
12. Campisi C, Boccardo F, Tacchella M. Reconstructive microsurgery of lymph vessels. *Microsurgery* 1995;16:161–6.

American Cancer Society Lymphedema Workshop

Supplement to **Cancer**

Imaging Techniques in the Management and Prevention of Posttherapeutic Upper Limb Edemas

Pierre Bourgeois, M.D., Ph.D.[1]
Oliver Leduc, P.T.[2]
Albert Leduc, Ph.D.[2]

[1] Nuclear Medicine Service Institut Jules Bordet and C.H.U. St. Pierre, Brussels, Belgium.

[2] Academic Department, Physical Therapy, Free University of Brussels, Brussels, Belgium.

BACKGROUND. Upper limb edema remains the most frequent complication after treatments for breast carcinoma. Various imaging techniques can be used to prevent these complications, to manage them, and to diagnose the possible lymphonodal evolution that may underlie these events. In the present paper, these techniques are reviewed.

METHODS. Based on clinical experience as well as on the data from the literature, these imaging techniques are presented, and their contributions are analyzed.

RESULTS. The pre- and post-operative imaging and research techniques of the so-called sentinel nodes (using blue dye, and/or lymphoscintigraphy, and/or gamma probe) appear to be very promising for defining patients in whom axillary node clearance either might be avoided or is indicated. Lymphoscintigraphic investigations also can be used after surgery and/or radiation therapy to define patients who either are at risk to develop upper limb edema or present with latent edema. In patients with clinically obvious edema, even if it is limited, lymphoscintigraphic techniques can provide a morphologic and functional definition of the condition. Venous echo Doppler can be used when abnormalities of the venous return are suspected. In diagnosing the lymphonodal evolution of the disease, techniques like immunoscintigraphy, positron emission tomography (using 18-fluoro-2-deoxy-D-glucose), X-ray computed tomography, and nuclear magnetic resonance imaging can contribute.

CONCLUSIONS. Various imaging techniques can be used to prevent and/or to manage the upper limb edema that may complicate the treatment(s) of the patients with breast carcinoma. *Cancer* 1998;83:2805–13.
© *1998 American Cancer Society.*

KEYWORDS: breast carcinoma, upper limb edema, imaging, lymphoscintigraphy, axillary node, sentinel node.

Posttherapeutic upper limb edema (PT-ULE) remains one of the most frequent complications for patients who are treated for breast carcinoma. In the present paper, imaging techniques are reviewed that can be used to prevent the appearance of such complications, to manage these situations, and to diagnose the lymphonodal evolution of the cancerous disease that may underlie these events.

Imaging Techniques for the Prevention of PT-ULE
Imaging techniques to avoid unnecessary axillary dissections or to limit the dissection

Because axillary dissection is the main cause for the appearance of ULE, the best way to avoid the "consequence" is to limit the "cause." Indeed, axillary node dissection might be said usefull only in cases where nodes are invaded upon anatomopathological (AP) examination (AP positive); in fact, and a priori, from 20% to 60–90% of patients

Presented at the American Cancer Society Lymphedema Workshop, New York, New York, February 20–22, 1998.

Address for reprints: Pierre Bourgeois, M.D., Ph.D., Nuclear Medicine Service, C.H.U. St. Pierre, 290 rue Haute, B-1000, Brussels, Belgium.

Received July 2, 1998; accepted August 20, 1998.

(according to their clinical T and N staging). Any technique that provides a preoperative diagnosis of the patient with AP-negative axilla might then help to avoid "unnecessary" axillary nodes clearance.

Ultrasonography of the axilla

Several authors have analyzed the contribution of ultrasonography in the preoperative staging of the axilla in breast carcinoma.[1-9] The positive predictive value of the technique usually is high (82% or more), but figures as low as 66%[2] or 69%[5] have been reported. On the other hand, the overall sensitivities of ultrasonography appear to be insufficient. Usually, they are between 63% and 73%, but values as low as 56% or as high as 89% were reported by De Freitas et al.[4] (n = 115) and by Ernst et al.[3] (n = 127), respectively. Furthermore, in small tumors (n = 39), Hergan et al.[8] reported that they found only two out of four cases with positive axillary nodes.

Immunoscintigraphy and the axillary nodes

A number of investigators have evaluated the use of breast carcinoma specific monoclonal antibodies in the staging of the axilla.[10-17] The studies *using the intravenous route* uniformly report a sensitivity lower for the detection of the axillary lymph node metastases (0–59%) than for that of primary breast carcinoma. *After subcutaneous injections,* the results appear to be better: The reported sensitivities range from 73.6% to 100%, and specificities are higher than 75%. However, published series are small (from 9 to 19 cases with positive nodes and from 9 to 54 cases with negative nodes).

Technetium-99m sestamibi mammoscintigraphy and the axillary nodes

Technetium-99m sestamibi (99mTc-MIBI) mammoscintigraphy has been proposed to detect and evaluate patients with primary breast carcinoma. Preliminary data suggest that this technique also is useful in the diagnosis of the metastatic axillary node involvement.[18,19] However, the last paper by Taillefer et al.[20] appears somewhat disappointing. Indeed, their sensitivity in detecting positive axillas was 79.2% (34 of 48), and their specificity was 84.6% (44 of 52). Their positive and negative predictive values were 82.6% (38 of 46) and 81.55% (44 of 54), respectively. The analysis of their data also shows that they detected only 33.3% of patients with a single positive node in the axilla (n = 9) and 75% of patients with two invaded nodes (n = 8).

Positron emission tomography using Fluorine-18-fluoro-2-deoxy-D-glucose (FDG) and the axillary nodes

In 1993, Adler et al.[21] reported a first series with 20 patients. Their sensitivity in the evaluation of the axilla

was 90% (9 of 10), and their negative predictive value was 91% (10 of 11). Later, in 50 patients,[22] they confirmed these figures with percentages equal to 95%.

However, Avril et al.[23] reported lower results, with a sensitivity of 79% (24 of 29) and a negative predictive value of 84% (26 of 31). Those authors also mentioned that among, their pT1 patients (n = 18), their sensitivity was only 33% (2 of 6). Holle et al.[24] also reported a series of 50 patients with a very low sensitivity, only 58%; however, only 12 patients in fact had AP positive axilla.

Recently, Crippa et al.[25] also reported their results of the prospective evaluation of Fluorine-18-FDG positron emission tomography (PET) for the presurgical staging of the axilla in breast carcinoma (n = 68). Their overall diagnostic accuracy was good (89%), but their sensitivity in clinically negative axilla was only 70%. Furthermore, the analysis of the presented data shows that three out of their five clinical T1N0 patients with AP positive axilla had micrometastasis and that two out of these three patients were negative upon PET.

Diagnostic lymphoscintigraphy

Several authors[26-35] have tried to use lymphoscintigraphy preoperatively and *in a diagnostic way.* Their results, based on small series, are disappointing and cannot be compared. Indeed, the products used as well as the sites of injection(s) (intramammary, peritumoral, subareolar, at the level of the arm) are variable. Furthermore, the images appear somewhat difficult to interpretate. For instance, MacLean and Ege[35] used 99mTc antimony sulphide colloid (a product that is no longer commercially available, at least in Europe) and, in 62 patients, injected their tracer into the first interdigital space of each hand. They classified their pictures as "definitely abnormal" (n = 14), "probably abnormal" (n = 12), "probably normal" (n = 13), and "definitely normal" (n = 23). The percentages of cases with positive nodes in these groups, respectively, were 93%, 58%, 38%, and 30%.

Lymphoscintigraphy (and blue dye) to define the sentinel node(s)

The use of lymphoscintigraphy, not as a way to diagnose the invasion of the axilla, but *to define the node(s)* (the sentinel nodes, SN) *at risk as positive* is more attractive. The concept was introduced in 1977 by Cabanas for penile carcinomas.[36] The SN is defined as the first lymph node in a regional lymphatic basin that receives the lymph from a primary tumor. This node is the first one encountered by tumor cells metastasing through lymph vessels and in which these cells may harbor and develop as micro- or macrometastases.

The histological status of the SN when it is resected selectively should then predict the status of all other subsequent nodes. The validity of the concept has been well established in melanoma, and the research and biopsy of the SN is now part of the surgical management of these clinically N0 carcinomas. When the SN is negative upon AP examination, no additional nodal resection is performed.

In breast carcinoma, the concept has been evaluated by several authors,[37-44] and results (from the first large series, with n = or >100) are promising and very encouraging. In 163 women and after subdermal and paratumoral injection of 99mTc-labeled human serum albumine colloid particles, Veronesi et al.[41] were successful in all but three patients in delineating the axillary SN. Their accuracy (status of the whole axilla well defined by the results of the SN) was 97.5% overall, but it was 100% when they considered their 45 patients with tumors less than 1.5 cm in greatest dimension. Their negative predictive value (n = 79) was 95%.

After intramammary and peritumoral injections, Giuliano et al.[39] were successful in delineating the axillary SN in 100 of 107 patients. Their overall accuracy and negative predictive value (n = 58) were 100%, and six of the seven patients in which no SN was observed had negative axilla.

Imaging techniques to define preoperatively the patients at risk for developing ULE

Several results suggest that, in patients who develop PT-ULE, some general and underlying lymphatic system disease might preexist and, perhaps, be identified. Carena et al.,[45] in a small series, have analyzed the functional lymphoscintigraphic data obtained at the level of the contralateral, nonedematous limbs of patients with monolateral ULE. Compared with a control group, their patients were significantly decreased. Investigating 428 patients with lymphoscintigraphy and prior to surgery, Pecking et al.[46] found that the functional index was abnormal in 32 patients (7.48% of the population) and reported that 27 of these 32 patients (84.4%) developed clinical edema by 34 months after surgery and radiotherapy.

Postoperative and preradiotherapy imaging techniques to define the patients at risk for developing ULE

In the literature, there are data[35,47] about the postoperative investigation of the upper limb lymphatic system, but, usually, they do not relate to the problem of PT-ULE. The systematic postoperative and preradiotherapeutic investigation of the axilla and of lymphatic drainage of the upper limbs was proposed more than 15 years ago by our group.[48-50] Performed at the same time as the lymphoscintigraphic investigation of the internal mammary chains (in which prognostic value is well established), the technique demonstrates and differentiates the nodes at the level of the axillas that receive lymph from the thoracic wall (on images obtained 2–3 hours after subcutaneous injection of the labeled tracer into the fifth or sixth intercostal space on the anterior axillary line) and/or from the upper limb (on images obtained 2–3 hours after subcutaneous injection of the tracer into the first interdigital space of each hand). Our studies (performed on large populations of patients who had been submitted to complete axillary nodes clearance) have demonstrated[51] that 1) the dissection could be called complete (operated axilla scintigraphically "empty") in only one-third of the patients who had been submitted to a so-called full dissection of the axilla (the mean number of axillary nodes found upon AP examination was 17); 2) such situations vary with the experience of the surgeons; and 3) the lymphatic drainage of the upper arm was "interrupted" (no axillary nodes was visualized after the interdigital injection) in 29.3% of patients (n = 965).

In one multivariate analysis,[51] three variables appeared to affect independently the fact that no axillary nodes were visualized after the interdigital injection (Id− situation): the delay after surgery (increased frequency of axillary node visualization for patients investigated more than 90 days after surgery, suggesting lymphatic collateralization or recovery with times); the age of the patients (the patients older than 60 years presented Id− situations more frequently); and the number of invaded nodes at the AP examination upon axillary dissection (more Id− in patients who presented more than three positive axillary nodes positive, suggesting that some Id− cases, in fact, were negative, because nodes were present in the axilla after surgery but were invaded).

With regard to the problem of PT-ULE, we might then demonstrate[51] that 1) the surgical interruption of upper limb lymphatic drainage pathways appeared in multivariate analysis as the most powerful predictor for the appearance of one ULE; in fact, the patients with such a condition had a relative risk (to develop ULE) 1.6 higher than the other patients and the actuarial cumulative percentage of ULE observed at 3 years was 33% for these patients (vs. 20% for other patients; $P < 0.0001$ using the log rank test comparing the two curves of events); 2) irradiation of the axilla and/or of the supraclavicular region also appeared as one independent variable (it is a classical notion that radiotherapy after surgery increases the frequency of ULE); however 3) surprisingly, in our analysis, the patients who were irradiated later had less frequency of ULE (even when previous factors were taken into account), and the observation remained as independent variable in one multivariate analysis.

Postoperative lymphoscintigraphic investigation of the upper limb in patients who received surgery of the axilla helps to define the patients at greatest risk to develop ULE later, especially if early radiotherapy also is planned. Such patients might be managed more carefully than others and can be informed of their risk.

However, our results concern patients who received to "full" axillary node dissection (the three levels of Berg and the apex), and it might be argued that, today, surgeons merely perform dissections that are limited to levels I and II. In that regard, it should be mentioned that Kett et al.[52] have performed radiological lymphography of the breast and the upper limb, and they observed that the two lymphatic systems connected in the upper segment of level II. Thus, the lymphatic drainage of the upper limb very probably is not spared in all cases by such "limited" surgeries.

Imaging techniques to define "latent" lymphedema

Using lymphoscintigraphy, Pecking et al.[46] found that, after surgery and radiotherapy, nearly all of their patients had one abnormal functional index (FI; FI <90%) and that the FI was severely depressed (≤70%) in 8.45% of patients (all with clinical edema). They also mention that, at that stage (after surgery and radiotherapy), 21% of the population presented with clinical edema, and 24% presented with preclinical edema. These values, respectively, changed to 33% and 9% 34 months later, suggesting that some patients with preclinical edema and abnormal FI (unfortunately, not specified in Pecking's paper) developed clinically obvious ULE.

Imaging Techniques for the Evaluation of PT-ULE
Imaging techniques to evaluate the lymphatic condition

The best way to evaluate the condition of lymphatic system in the upper limbs is to use lymphoscintigraphic techniques.[53–65] After subcutaneous (or intradermal) injections of 99mTc-labeled colloidal particles in one (or more) interdigital space(s), dynamic as well as static images may be obtained at various levels (the forearms, the elbows, the arms, and the axillas) and under various standardized conditions (during and/or after various periods of rest, during and/or after exercise, after various periods of normal activity). These investigations provide morphologic and functional information about the superficial lymphatic system in the upper limbs. The functional or numerical values obtained may be expressed with reference to the patient's contralateral arm (considered as normal) and/or with reference to the data obtained from a control population.

With regard to the morphologic information, upper limb lymphoscintigraphy may show that the tracer does not appear at the level of *both* forearms in resting conditions, thus suggesting one general lymphatic insufficiency; that the tracer (usually with exercise) does not flow through lymphatic vessels but through subdermis (progression through subdermal collateralization); that the tracer flows first through lymphatic vessels but, later, flows back into the subdermis when reaching the axilla or one level of blockade (dermal backflow); that dermal backflow may be limited to one part of the upper limb; that the tracer is blocked at the level of the axilla or more distally; that axillary and/or supraclavicular lymph nodes are present and receive lymph from the upper limb; and that lymphatic collateralization pathways are present and are naturally opened at the level of the shoulder (the so-called "Mascagni's" pathway), through the axilla, from the operated axilla toward the contralateral axilla, from the axilla toward the homolateral internal mammary nodes, and through the chest wall.

From a functional point of view, various parameters may be calculated (in various conditions): the time for the tracer to reach the axilla; the lymphatic "speed"; the time to reach the half-maximum activity at the level of the axilla (when axillary nodes are present); the percentage of lymphatic extraction (in fact, the disappearance of the tracer) at the level of the injected sites; the activity in the liver (when only the edematous upper limb, is injected), which is representative of the lymph leaving the upper limb and reaching the the great circulation; and the activity in the limb, which is representative of the lymph stasis. These morphologic data and functional parameters can be and have been integrated into functional indices by several authors. The morphologic indices obtained under standardized conditions as well as the functional data allow classification of ULE into morphofunctional categories.

For instance, based on the extraction (disappearance) of the labeled tracer at the sites of injection (analyzed 1, 3, 6, 9, and 24 hours later), we proposed to classify the PT-ULE functionally as "lymphatic predominant" (or "pure" lymphedema), "venous predominant" (the "venedema" cases), or as presenting a "mixed pattern" (the "venolymphedema" cases). Indeed, we demonstrated in one series of 50 patients with unilateral PT-ULE that 16 had values at the level of their edematous limb less than 50% of their normal limb values (group 1), 14 had values between 50% and 100% of their contralateral arm (group 2), and 20 had extraction values by their edematous arm higher than those observed at the level of their nonedematous limb (group 3).

Upper limb radionuclide phlebographies could be performed therafter in 25 patients (ten in group 1, ten in group 3, and five in group 2). In all but one-half of the patients in group 1, abnormalities of the venous return were demonstrated (complete blockade of the axillary vein with collateralization, stenosis of the axillary vein, axillary vein not visualized but venous return through the cephalic vein, delayed venous return). Pecking et al.[53] also noted that their patients with associated abnormalities of the venous return had lymphatic flow rate indicies higher than others.

Furthermore, we also were able to demonstrate that the most voluminous edemas were associated with the absence of nodal visualization in the axilla. In their series, Pecking et al.[53] found this situation in 62% of their patients. This percentage must be compared with the relative risk (1.6) for developing ULE[51] that we had found for our patients with no axillary nodes visualized postoperatively compared with others.

These investigations and their results may have therapeutic implications: They may "direct" the hand of the physical therapist, who will mobilize the zones of lymph stasis; the patients with venedema will have to wear stockings to maintain the effects of the treatments; and they show that lymph nodes and/or lymph vessels are present with good flow and that they may be used to perform anastomosis to veins. Several authors have reported their use as a way to evaluate treatments as well as to follow their patients.[61–65]

Imaging techniques to evaluate venous return abnormalities

Edema of the arm after breast carcinoma surgery and radiotherapy may be associated with and/or secondary to a venous impairment. The reported frequencies of these venous abnormalities (VA) at the level of the edematous upper limbs are highly variable. They probably depend on the population analyzed (with variables, such as the kind of surgery performed, the postoperative complications, the irradiation of the axilla, the importance of the ULE, its duration, etc., taken into account), on the criteria applied to define a venous impairment, and on the technique used. By using radionuclide phlebography, as discussed above, we observed VA in 20 (80%) of our cases (n = 25) but axillary vein thrombosis in only two patients (8%). Using radiologic phlebography, Pecking et al.[53] observed VA in 24% of their patients (18 of 75). Those authors also noted that the patients with VA had ULE more voluminous than the patients without VA. In a small series, Cambria et al.[57] noted that 2 of the 14 patients (14%) who underwent venous evaluation

(venography in nine, noninvasive studies in five) had evidence of venous *obstruction*. Using ultrasonography in a series of 50 patients, Ghabboun et al.[66] found venous *thrombosis* in ten cases (20%). Three venous thrombosis cases were acute, and the others were old, but, among the remaining seven patients, only two were diagnosed at the time of the investigation. They also noted that thickening of the walls of the axillary and subclavian veins was present in 30% of patients. Using Doppler flowmetry, Zanolla et al.[67] investigated 240 patients who received modified mastectomy or conservative surgery for breast carcinoma. Postoperatively, they found important abnormalities of the venous return in ten cases, or only 4% (thrombophlebitis or extrinsic compression of the axillary or humeral vein). They mention that these abnormalities caused the immediate appearance of ULE, the size of which was much greater than that of the solely lymphatic ULE (which appeared later). They also noted that, in 80% of the patients with abnormal Doppler flowmetry, the edema usually was medium and/or large in size and tended to persist.

Phlebographic investigations of the upper limbs, radiological or radioisotopic, might be proposed and performed in patients with PT-ULE. However, the best way to evaluate the venous return with certainty is to use Doppler flowmetry. This technique enables us not only to demonstrate morphologic abnormalities but also to analyze venous flow functionally through the axilla under the various conditions of daily life situations that may influence the pathophysiology of the edema.

Imaging techniques to evaluate other tissular parameters and/or modifications

If lymphoscintigraphic investigations and ultrasonography usually are sufficient to evaluate the lymphatic and venous changes in PT-ULE morphologically and functionally, other imaging techniques sometimes may be useful: Laser-Doppler to evaluate microcirculation,[68] X-ray computed tomography,[69] or magnetic nuclear resonance[70] (with or without injection of contrast media). These two latter techniques can be used to evaluate water infiltration or the fatty of fibrotic nature of tissular changes in the edematous limb, or they can be used to evaluate precisely the thickness and density of the skin and the subcutis. Much cheaper than the other techniques, plain xeroradiography[69] has been used to evaluate the skin and the subcutis, and[71] biphotonic absorbtiometry has been used to study the lean and fat mass of PT-ULE.

PT-ULE and the Lymph Nodal Evolution of the Cancerous Disease

Among many factors, the locoregional evolution of the cancerous disease involving the axillary nodes and/or lymphatic vessels may explain the appearance of PT-ULE. Such an evolution may be clinically obvious in several cases (palpable lymph nodes). However, usually, it is "silent" and difficult to demonstrate. In a retrospective review of our data,[72] clinically obvious nodal relapses (NR) were observed in association with PT-ULE in only 10% of patients (22 of 237). These NR with PT-ULE patients, however, were found more frequently (10 of 36 or 27.8% of the RX-N++ patients) when no irradiation of the nodal basins was performed (RX− patients; 11 of 69 vs. 11 of 168) and when more than 3 nodes had been found positive at the AP in the axillary piece of dissection (N++ patients; 15 of 90 or 16.7% vs. 7 of 147). In the group without PT-ULE, the nodal relapses were observed less frequently, respectively, in 19.6% of the RX-N++ patients and in 12.7% of the N++ patients. The patients with ULE who presented more than three axillary AP-positive nodes and who were not irradiated on their nodal basins, thus, may represent a group in which it is justified to search for a clinical or "silent" lymph nodal evolution of the disease. Another situation in which such research might be performed is the patient with ULE (increasing or not, that does not respond to applied treatments) with no generalization and with increased or increasing tumoral markers. X-ray computed tomography and ultrasonography may be used in such cases, and their values as well as their limitations (size and density of the lesions) are well known. More attractive is the technique of immunoscintigraphies with 99mTc- or 111In-labeled monoclonal antibodies against mammary carcinomatous antigens. Indeed, it was reported to be successful in 1989 by Pecking et al.[73] but in a limited series of such patients. The interest in the technique is supported by another, more recent report. In a series of 51 evaluable patients (15 with primary breast carcinoma and 38 with metastatic carcinoma at the time of the investigation), McQuarrie et al.[74] mentioned that radioimmunoscintigraphy (RIS) was be positive in 42 (84%) of the 50 "locoregional" diseases. The technique seems to be sensitive, but its specificity remains to be established in such cases. With one sensitivity of 100% (8 of 8) for the lymph node localizations in patients with recurrent or metastatic breast carcinoma,[75] PET using 2-(Fluorine-18)-FDG seems as attractive as RIS. However, the reported specificity is only 13% (or 60% according to the chosen score).

Conclusions

To conclude and to summarize the present paper, the following imaging techniques seem interesting and can be used in patients with carcinoma of the breast, either to prevent PT-ULE or to manage it. The preoperative lymphoscintigraphic demonstration of the axillary SN with the peroperative use of gamma probe (and of blue dye) to selectively dissect it; if the SN is negative upon AP examination, then unnecessary lymph node dissection can be avoided. Imaging techniques, such as PET using Fluorine-18-FDG, (lympho)-immunoscintigraphies, (mammo-)scintigraphies with 99mTc-MIBI, or ultrasonography, can be taken into consideration only when they are positive (expecially in small tumors with clinically negative axilla, their sensitivities in detecting positive node(s) harboring mainly micrometastases have seemed to be insufficient). When axillary node dissection (complete or even limited) is indicated and performed, the postoperative lymphoscintigraphic investigation of the upper limbs is indicated. The technique will allow to define the cases where the surgery has interrupted the normal lymphatic pathways draining the limb. These patients must be managed more carefully than others, and they represent a population in which some policies of prevention should be applied (or tested).

When the patient presents with ULE, the following imaging techniques should be applied: 1) one lymphoscintigraphic investigation of the upper limb(s) (combining static and dynamic imagings, morphological and functional data); 2) one investigation of the axillary vein (when indicated by the clinic or when lymphoscintigraphy suggests the venous or mixed pattern of the ULE); 3) when it is suspected, any technique allowing the demonstration of the lymph nodal evolution of the disease in the axilla; and 4) biphotonic absorbtiometry to evaluate the fat and lean mass. These techniques will characterize the edema morphologically and functionally. Sometimes, they will direct the treatments to be applied, and, in many cases, they will allow a good assessment of the therapeutic responses.

REFERENCES

1. Bruneton JN, Caramella E, Hery M, Aubanel D, Manzino JJ, Picard JL. Axillary lymph node metastases in breast cancer: preoperative detection with US. *Radiology* 1986;158:325–6.
2. Tate JJT, Lewis V, Arehcer T, Guyer PG, Royle T, Taylor I. Ultrasound detection of axillary nodes metastases in breast cancer. *Eur J Surg Oncol* 1989;15:139–41.
3. Ernst R, Weber A, Bauer KH, Friemann J, Zumtobel V. Perioperative ultrasound imaging of the breast in breast cancer. *Zentrabl Chir* 1990;115:963–75.

4. De Freitas R Jr., Costa MV, Schneider SV, Nicolau MA, Marussi E. Accuracy of ultrasound and clinical examination in the diagnosis of axillary node metastases in breast cancer. *Eur J Surg Oncol* 1991;17:240–4.

5. Tohnosu N, Okuyama K, Koide Y, Kikuchi T, Awano T, Matsubara H, et al. A comparison between ultrasonography and mammography, computed tomography and digital subtraction angiography for the detection of breast cancers. *Surg Today* 1993;28:704–10.

6. Walsh JS, Dixon JM, Chetty U, Paterson D. Colour doppler studies of axillary nodes metastases in breast carcinoma. *Clin Radiol* 1994;49:189–91.

7. Vaidya JS, Vyas JJ, Thakur MH, Khandelwal KC, Mittra I. Role of ultrasonography to detect axillary node involvement in operable breast cancer. *Eur J Surg Oncol* 1996;22:140–3.

8. Hergan K, Haid A, Zimmermann G, Oser W. Preoperative axillary ultrasound in breast carcinoma: value of the method in clinical practice. *Ultraschall Med* 1996;17:14–7.

9. Bonnema J, VanGeel AN, VanOoijen B, Mali SP, Tjian SL, Henzen-Logmans SC, Schmitz PI, Wiggers T. Ultrasound guided aspiration biopsy for detection of non palpable axillary node metastases in breast cancer patients: new diagnostic method. *World J Surg* 1997;21:270–4.

10. DeLand F, Kim E, Corgan R. Axillary lymphoscintigraphy in radio-immunodetection of carcino-embryogenic antigen in breast cancer" *J Nucl Med* 1979;20:1243–50.

11. Thompson CH, Stacker SA, Salehi N. Immunoscintigraphy for detection of lymph node metastases from breast cancer. *Lancet* 1984;2:1245–7.

12. Mandeville R, Pateisky N, Philipp K, Kubista E, Dumas F, Grouix B. Immunolymphoscintigraphy of axillary lymph node metastases in breast cancer patients using monoclonal antibodies: first clinical findings. *Anticancer Res* 1986;6: 1257–64.

13. Tjandra JJ, Russel IS, Collins JP, Andrews JT, Lichtenstein M, Bins D, MacKenzie IFC. Immunolymphoscintigraphy for the detection of lymph node metastases from breast cancer. *Cancer Res* 1989;49:1600–8.

14. Tjandra JJ, Sacks NPM, Thompson CH. The detection of axillary lymph node metastases from breast cancer by radiolabeled monoclonal antibodies: a prospective study. *Br J Cancer* 1989;59:291–302.

15. Kairemo KJA. Immunolymphoscintigraphy with 99mTc-labeled monoclonal antibody (BW431/26) reacting with carcinoembryonic antigen in breast cancer. *Cancer Res* 1990; 50:949–54.

16. Lamki LM, Buzdar AU, Singletary SL. Indium-111-labeled B72.3 monoclonal antibody in the detection and staging of breast cancer: a Phase I study. *J Nucl Med* 1991;32:1326–32.

17. Taylor JL, Taylor DL, Lowry C. Radioimmunoscintigraphy of metastatic breast carcinoma. *Eur J Surg Oncol* 1992;18:57–63.

18. Taillefer R, Robidoux A, Lambert R, Turpin S, Laperrière J. Technetium-99m sestamibi prone scintimammography to detect primary breast cancer and axillary node involvement. *J Nucl Med* 1995;36:1758–65.

19. Lamm WWM, Yang WT, Stewart IET, Metreweli C, King W. Detection of axillary lymph node metastases in breast carcinoma by technetium-99m sestamibi breast scintigraphy, ultrasound and conventional mammography. *Eur J Nucl Med* 1996;23:498–503.

20. Taillefer R, Robidoux A, Turpin S, Lambert R, Cantin J, Léveillé J. Metastatic axillary lymph node technetium-99m-

21. MIBI imaging in primary breast cancer. *J Nucl Med* 1998;39: 459–64.

21. Adler LP, Crowe JP, Al-Kaisi NK, Sunshine JL. Evaluation of breast masses and axillary lymph nodes with 2-(Fluorine-18)-fluoro-2-deoxy-D-glucose PET. *Radiology* 1993;187:743–50.

22. Adler LP, Failhaber PF, Schnur KC, Al-Kasi NL, Shenk RR. Axillary lymph node metastases: screening with (F-18)2-deoxy-2-Fluoro-d-glucose (FDG) PET. *Radiology* 1997;203: 323–7.

23. Avril N, Dose J, Janicke F, Ziegler S, Romer W, Weber W, Herz M, Nathrath W, Graeff H, Schwaiger M. Assessment of axillary lymph node involvement in breast cancer patients with positron emission tomography using radiolabeled 2-(Fluorine-18)-fluoro-2-deoxy-D-glucose. *J Natl Cancer Inst* 1996;88:1204–9.

24. Holle LH, Trampert L, Lung-Kurt S, Villena-Heinsen CE, Pischel W, Schmidt S, Oberhausen E. Investigation of breast tumours with fluorine-18-fluorodeoxyglucose and SPECT. *J Nucl Med* 1996;37:615–22.

25. Crippa F, Agresti R, Seregni E, Greco M, Pascali C, Bogni A, Chiesa C, DeSanctis V, Delledonne V, Salvadori B, Leutner M, Bombardieri E. Prospective evaluation of Fluorine-18-FDG PET in presurgical staging of the axilla in breast cancer. *J Nucl Med* 1998;39:4–8.

26. Agwunobi TC, Boak JL. Diagnosis of malignant breast disease by axillary lymphoscintigraphy: a preliminary report. *Br J Surg* 1979;3:379–83.

27. Black RB, Merrick MV, Taylor TV. Prediction of axillary metastases in breast cancer by lymphoscintigraphy. *Lancet* 1980;2:15–17.

28. Christensen B, Blichert-Toft M, Siemssen OJ, Nielsen SL. Reliability of axillary lymph node scintiphotography in suspected carcinoma of the breast. *Br J Surg* 1980;67: 667–8.

29. Boak JL, Ingoldby CJH, Nathan BE, Meyers G. The role of axillary lymphoscintigraphy in the diagnosis of breast cancer. *Clin Oncol* 1981;7:45–52.

30. Black RB, Merrick MV, Taylor TV, Forrest APM. Lymphoscintigraphy cannot diagnose breast cancer. *Br J Surg* 1981; 68:145–6.

31. Gabelle P, Comet M, Bodin JP, Dupré A, Carpentier E, Bolla M, Swiercz P. Mammary lymphatic scintiscans by intratumoral injection in the assessment of breast cancer. *Nouv Presses Med* 1981;10:3067–70.

32. Osborne MP, Payna JH, Richardson VJ, McReady VR, Ryman BE. The preoperative detection of axillary lymph nodes metastases in breast cancer by isotope imaging. *Br J Surg* 1983; 70:141–4.

33. Hill NS, Ege GN, Greyson ND, et al. Predicting by lymphoscintigraphy of nodal metastases in breast cancer. *Can J Surg* 1983;26:507–9.

34. Mazzeo F, Accurso A, Petrella G, Capuano S, Maurelli L, Clenetano L, Squame G, Salvatore M. Preoperative axillary lymphoscintigraphy in breast cancer: experience with subareolar injection of 99mTc-nanocolloidal albumin. *Nucl Med Comm* 1986;7:5–16.

35. McLean RG, Ege GN. Prognostic value of axillary lymphoscintigraphy in breast carcinoma patients. *J Nucl Med* 1986; 27:1116–24.

36. Cabanas RM. An approach for the treatment of penile carcinoma. *Cancer* 1977;39:456–66.

37. Krag DN, Weaver DL, Alex JC, Fairbanks JT. Surgical resection and radiolocalization of the sentinel lymph nodes in breast cancer using a gamma probe. *Surg Oncol* 1993;2:335–40.

38. Albertini JJ, Lyman OH, Cox C, Yeatman T, Balducci L, Ku NN, Shivers S, Berman C, Wells K, Rapaport D, Shons A, Horton J, Greenberg H, Nicosia S, Clark R, Cantor A, Reintgen D. Lymphatic mapping and sentinel node biopsy in the patient with breast cancer. *JAMA* 1996;276:1818–22.

39. Giuliano A, Jones R, Brennan M, Statman R. Sentinel Lymphadenectomy in breast cancer. *J Clin Oncol* 1997;15:2345–50.

40. Turner R, Ollilla D, Krasne D, Giuliano A. Histopathologic validation of the sentinel lymph node hypothesis for breast carcinoma. *Ann Surg* 1997;226:271–8.

41. Veronesi U, Paganelli G, Galimberti V, Viale G, Zurrida S, Bedoni M, Costa A, De Cicco C, Geraghty JG, Luini A, Sacchini V, Veronesi P. Sentinel-node biopsy to avoid axillary dissection in breast cancer with clinically negative lymphnodes. *Lancet* 1997;349:1864–7.

42. El-Shirbiny AM, Yeh S, Cody HS, Borgen PI, Larson SM. Scintigraphic identification of sentinel lymph node in breast cancer [abstract]. *Eur J Nucl Med* 1997;24:892.

43. Gulec SA, Moffat FL, Serafini AN, Sfakianakis GN, Allen L, Boggs J, Escobedo D, Sundaram M, Boyle M, Livingstone A, Krag D. Sentinel node localization in patients with breast cancer [abstract]. *J Nucl Med* 1997;38:33P.

44. Pijpers R, Meijer S, Hoekstra OS, Collet GJ, Comans EF, Boom RP, VanDiest PJ, Teule JG. Impact of lymphoscintigraphy on sentinel node identification with technetium-99m-colloidal albumin in breast cancer. *J Nucl Med* 1997;38:366–8.

45. Carena M, Baiardi P, Saponaro M, Mazzoieni MC, Rossi G, Paroni G, Aprile C. Scintigraphic evaluation of predisposition to post-mastectomy lymphedema. In: Progress in Lymphology XIII. Cluzan RV, et al., editors. Berlin: Springer-Verlag, 1992:325–6.

46. Pecking AP, Floiras JL, Rouessé J. Upper limb lymphedema's frequency in patients treated by conservative therapy in breast cancer. *Lymphology* 1996;29(Suppl):293–6.

47. Muller RP, Tillkorn H, Peters PE. Lymphography of the upper limb following radical axillary lymph node dissection" In: Progress in Lymphology. Weissleider H, Bartos V, Clodius L, Málek P, editors. Prague: Avicenum Czechoslovsk Medical Press, 1981:226–9.

48. Bourgeois P, Fruhling J, Henry J. Postoperative axillary lymphoscintigraphy in the management of breast cancer. *Int J Radiat Oncol Biol Phys* 1983;9:29–32.

49. Fruhling J, Bourgeois P. Axillary lymphoscintigraphy: current status in the treatment of breast cancer. *CRC Crit Rev Oncol Hematol* 1983;1:1–20.

50. Mattheiem W, Bourgeois P, Delcorde A, Stegen M, Fruhling J. Axillary dissection in breast cancer revisited. *Eur J Surg Oncol* 1989;15:490–5.

51. Bourgeois P. Les investigations lymphoscintigraphiques post-opératoires des chaînes mammaires internes et des creux axillaires dans le bilan et le pronostic des cancers du sein (the postoperative investigations of the axilla and of the internal mammary chains in the management and prognosis of breast carcinomas). Thèse d'Agrégation de l'Enseignement Supérieur, Faculté de Médecine, Université Libre de Bruxelles. Brussels, Belgium: 1997.

52. Kett K, Szilagyi K, Clodius L. The value of combined lymphography in the diagnosis of lymph node metastases in breast cancer. In: Progress in lymphology XIII. Excerpta medica. Cluzan RV, et al., editors. Amsterdam: Elsevier Science Publishers, 1992:371–2.

53. Pecking AP, Firmin F, Rain JD, Desprez-Curely JP, Cluzan RV, Jacquillat C, Banzet P. Lymphoedeme post-chirurgical et radiothérapique des membres supérieurs: exploration par la lymphographie isotopique indirecte (lymphedema of the upper limb following surgery or radiotherapy: investigation by indirect radioactive lymphography). *Nouv Presse Méd* 1980;9:3349–51.

54. Kaplan WD, Slavin SA, Markisz JA, Laffin SM, Royal HD. Qualitative and quantitative upper extremity radionuclide lymphoscintigraphy [abstract]. *J Nucl Med* 1983;24:40.

55. Carena M, Campini R, Zelaschi G, Rossi G, Aprile C, Paroni G. Quantitative lymphoscintigraphy. *Eur J Nucl Med* 1988;14:88–92.

56. Weissleder H, Wielssleder R. Lymphedema: evaluation of qualitative and quantitative lymphoscintigraphy in 238 patients. *Radiology* 1988;167:729–35.

57. Cambria RA, Glovczki P, Naessens JA, Wahner HW. Noninvasive evaluation of the lymphatic system with lymphoscintigraphy: a prospective, semiquantitative analysis in 386 extremities. *J Vasc Surg* 1993;18:773–82.

58. Golucke PJ, Montgomery RA, Petronis JD, Minken SL, Peter BA, Williams GM. Lymphoscintigraphy to confirm the clinical diagnosis of lymphedema. *J Vasc Surg* 1989;10:306–12.

59. Kleinhans E, Baumeister RGH, Hahn D, Siuda S, Büll U, Moser E. Evaluation of transport kinetics in lymphoscintigraphy: follow-up study in patients with transplanted vessels. *Eur J Nucl Med* 1985;10:349–52.

60. Ter SE, Alavi A, Kim CK, Merli G. Lymphoscintigraphy: a reliable test for the diagnosis of lymphedema. *Clin Nucl Med* 1993;18:646–54.

61. De Groote M, Jonnart C, Puissant F, Buisset J, Schlikker E. Lymphoscintigraphic evaluation of the efficiency of manual lymphatic drainage. *Eur J Lymphol Rel Prob* 1992;3:85–7.

62. Verlooy H, Biscompte JP, Nieuborg L, Drent P, Schiepers C, Mortelmans L, De Roo M. Noninvasive evaluation of lymphovenous anastomosis in upper lymphedema: value of quantitative lymphoscintigraphic examinations. *Eur J Lymphol Rel Probl* 1997;6:27–33.

63. Weiss M, Baumeister RGH, Tatsch K, Hahn K. Lymphoscintigraphy and semiquantitative evaluation of lymph drainage for long-term follow-up in patients with autogenous lymph vessel transplantation. *Eur J Lymphol Rel Probl* 1997;6:34–37.

64. Ferrandez JC, Serin D, Vinot JM. Lymphoscintigraphic assessment of manual lymphatic drainage: report of 47 observations. *Eur J Lymphol Rel Probl* 1997;6:38–46.

65. Vaqueiro M, Glowiczki P, Fischer J, Hollier LH. Lymphoscintigraphy in lymphedema: an aid to microsurgery. *J Nucl Med* 1986;27:1125–30.

66. Ghabboun S, Alliot F, Cluzan RV, Pascot M. Venous disorders in secondary upper limb lymphedema. *Lymphology* (suppl) 1998;31:519–21.

67. Zanolla R, Blandini MG, Balzarini A, Feria F, Pirovano C. Breast cancer: oedema post-axillary dissection. Is Doppler flowmetry evaluation predictive for edema? Are there precautionary therapies after surgery? In: Progress in lymphology XIII. Cluzan RV, editors. Berlin: Springer-Verlag, 1992:621–2.

68. Boccardo F, Tacchella M, Zilli A, Campisi C. Laser-Doppler evaluation in peripheral lymphedema. *Lymphology* (suppl) 1998;31:279–81.

69. Bruna J. Computerized tomography and xeroradiography in evaluation of oedemas. *Eur J Lymphol Rel Probl* 1991;2:1–4.

70. Unger EC, Baker MR. Role of magnetic resonance imaging in the evaluation of lymphedema and disease of the lymphatics. *Lymphology* 1994;27(Suppl):249–51.

71. Cluzan RV, Pecking A, Ruiz JC, Alliot F, Ghabboun S, Pascot M, Gachon-Lameyre V. Biphotonic aborbtiometry of the secundary upper limb lymphedema. *Lymphology* (suppl) 1998;31:296–8.

72. Bourgeois P. Nodal relapse(s) and lymphedema(s). In: Vascular medicine. Boccalon H, editor. Amsterdam: Elsevier Science Publisher, 1993:453–6.

73. Pecking A, Delorme G, Briere B. Exploration du lymphoedeme par les marqueurs biologiques [oral presentation]. Euromedicine, Montpellier, 1989.

74. McQuarrie SA, MacLean GD, Boniface GR, Golberg K, McEwan AJB. Radioimmunoscintigraphy in patients with breast adenocarcinoma using technetium-99-m labelled monoclonal antibody 170H.82: report of a Phase II study. *Eur J Nucl Med* 1997;24:381–9.

75. Moon DH, Maddahi J, Silverman DHS, Glaspy JA, Phelps ME, Hoh CK. Accuracy of whole-body fluorine-18-FDG PET for the detection of recurrent or metastatic breast cancer. *J Nucl Med* 1998;39:431–5.

American Cancer Society Lymphedema Workshop

*Supplement to **Cancer***

Precipitating Factors in Lymphedema: Myths and Realities

Stanley G. Rockson, M.D.

Lymphedema Center, Division of Cardiovascular Medicine, Stanford University School of Medicine, Stanford, California.

BACKGROUND. Lymphedema is an all too common occurrence following breast carcinoma therapy. Despite its prevalence, the predisposing factors to the development of this secondary form of lymphedema remain poorly understood.

METHODS. Several studies have addressed these questions and are reviewed here.

RESULTS. Treatment factors that appear to predispose to the late, subjective appearance of lymphedema include the extent of axillary surgery and exposure to high dose axillary radiotherapy, particularly when combined with surgical clearance of the axilla. Other pertinent patient factors may include the presence of hypertension and exposure to airline travel. Clinical features unrelated to the risk of lymphedema development include patient age; drug therapy; time interval to presentation, surgery, or radiotherapy to the breast; total dose of radiation; and menopausal status. The potential importance of concomitant venous abnormalities in these patients is worthy of consideration.

CONCLUSIONS. Breast carcinoma-related secondary lymphedema is an important subjective and functional problem for affected patients. Additional research into the predisposing factors to this common problem is likely to foster enhanced patient education and to produce more efficacious measures to control this disease. ***Cancer* 1998;83:2814–6.** © *1998 American Cancer Society.*

KEYWORDS: lymphedema, radiotherapy, cellulitis, venous obstruction.

Lymphedema of the upper extremity frequently can accompany or complicate the therapy of breast carcinoma. Although estimates of the frequency of this complication have varied to some degree,[1,2] it is not unreasonable to conjecture that, during the natural history of posttherapeutic breast carcinoma, perhaps 30% of patients might have clinical manifestations of impaired lymphatic function in the arm. Improvements in surgical and radiotherapeutic techniques apparently have reduced the incidence of lymphedematous complications; nevertheless, arm swelling appears to be an inevitable consequence of breast carcinoma therapy for substantial numbers of patients.

Significant confusion continues to surround the temporal behavior of this type of secondary lymphedema. The inability to identify reliably the precipitating factors that cause the lymphedema to appear or to worsen has served to foster fear and frustration in patients who are at risk by virtue of prior breast carcinoma therapy. Many of the patient education materials in current use continue to promulgate behavioral adaptations and modifications emanating from an unsubstantiated, empirically derived conception of the physical forces that govern the progression of lymphedema.[3] Such "dos-and-don'ts" (Table 1) have not changed appreciably in several generations of cancer therapy, and, unfortunately, few objective data have been accumu-

Presented at the American Cancer Society Lymphedema Workshop, New York, New York, February 20–22, 1998.

Address for reprints: Stanley G. Rockson, M.D., Assistant Professor of Medicine, Falk Cardiovascular Research Center, Stanford University School of Medicine, Stanford, CA 94305.

Received July 2, 1998; accepted August 20, 1998.

TABLE 1
"Dos and Don'ts" for Postmastectomy Patients[a]

Every effort must be made to avoid all cuts, scratches, pinpricks, hangnails, insect bites, burns, and strong detergents

Do not pick at or cut cuticles or hangnails

Do not dig in the garden or work near thorny plants

Do not reach into a hot oven

Do not permit injections, blood specimens, or blood pressure recordings in this arm

Do wear loose fitting rubber gloves when washing dishes

Do wear a thimble when sewing

Do apply a good lanolin-based hand cream often

Do contact your doctor if your arm appears red, warm, or unusually swollen

[a] See Nelson, 1966.[3]

TABLE 2
Factors Unrelated to the Late Development of Lymphedema[a]

Age

Drug therapy

Time interval since presentation

Surgery to the breast

Radiotherapy to the breast

Total dose of radiation

Menopausal status

Early lymphedema

[a] See Kissin et al., 1986.[4]

lated to validate the clinical recommendations. For example, patients often voice substantial concern about the acceptable limits for upper extremity exertion either in a recreational context or to support the activities of daily living; at this time, with a paucity of scientifically derived data, clinicians cannot answer such questions knowledgeably.

What, then, is known of the pertinent variables that influence the appearance of lymphedema in these patients? Fortunately, the careful scrutiny of more recent patient series has begun to dispel some long-cherished myths about treatment-derived, precipitating factors, and our comprehension of the potential role of coattendant morbidities has grown in a parallel fashion. Furthermore, some the treatment factors that might foster the ultimate development of upper extremity lymphedema seem to have become more readily identified.

To this end, the analysis by Kissin in 1986 of his series of 200 patients is quite instructive.[4] In this series, lymphedema was noted subjectively in 14% of the patients, yet measurement of the volume of the extremities yielded a much more substantial 25.5% incidence of arm swelling following the patients' carcinoma therapy. Treatment factors that predisposed significantly to the late, subjective appearance of lymphedema included the extent of axillary surgery ($P < 0.05$) and the exposure to axillary radiotherapy ($P < 0.001$), whereas the pathological node status seemed to bear no statistically significant relation to the lymphedematous complication. The highest incidence of late lymphedema was seen in the group of patients who had undergone both surgical clearance of the axilla and radiotherapy (38.3%). Of substantial additional interest is the list of patient factors that appear to be unrelated to the development of lymphedema: patient age, drug therapy, time interval since presentation, surgery or radiotherapy to breast,

total dose of radiation, menopausal status, and the early, postsurgical appearance of edema (Table 2).

A subsequently published study of 136 patients is similarly instructive.[1] In this series, once again, patient age did not appear to play a role nor did the requirement for surgery on the neurologically dominant side (a fact that might indirectly shed light on the role of exercise and muscular use of the involved extremity). Obesity, radiotherapy, and an oblique surgical incision were all unfavorable treatment factors. Of most predictive value for the development of lymphedema were the use of high dose axillary radiotherapy and a history of infection in the ipsilateral upper extremity (Table 2). Furthermore, the presence of hypertension in 51 of 130 patients seemed to predispose to development of lymphedema ($P < 0.005$), whereas other preexisting cardiovascular conditions predisposed not to lymphedema but to higher rates of subcutaneous fibrosis ($P < 0.002$).

One patient factor that often merits subjective patient commentary is the apparent temporal relation of airline travel to the appearance or exacerbation of lymphedema. This precipitant, in fact, has been evaluated objectively in the form of a prospective, questionnaire-driven analysis of precipitating factors in a large population of lymphedema patients.[5] Indeed, high incidence of new lymphedema and exacerbation of preexisting conditions were identified by these patients in association with the triggering event of air travel. It is conjectured that the problem may be attributable to a lowered cabin pressure that, in turn, exacerbates the lymphatic incompetence of the lymphostatic limb. The reduced contribution of muscular pumping in the involved extremity may contribute to the temporary obstruction of venous and lymphatic drainage.

Once lymphedema becomes established following breast carcinoma therapy, the temporal duration of the edematous state appears to represent an additional factor that will contribute to the likelihood of progression. In a study of 231 patients, it was observed that the lymphedema had a significant tendency to increase with time, both in grade and in quantity.[6] Although both patient age and the duration of lymphedema are significant influences, it is the latter that apparently is of greater importance. The inexorable tendency for lymphedema to progress has been emphasized by others as well.[7]

In an attempt to identify the modifiable, precipitating patient factors in lymphedema, it is important to remember the complex nature of the pathoanatomic derangement following breast carcinoma surgery. The potentially multifactorial nature of postmastectomy edema was well recognized by Halsted, who, in the early descriptions of his patient population, underscored the importance of infection and, at times, venous disruption as contributory features in the development of lymphedema after iatrogenic, surgical disruption of the lymphatic channels.[8] Since that time, the importance of the venous contribution to the edema in breast carcinoma patients has been debated and repeatedly reexplored. More recently, the question has been readdressed through the modality of color Doppler imaging of the upper extremity venous flow patterns.[9] In this study of 81 patients, over half had evidence of venous outflow obstruction; in fact, only 30% of the swollen arms had a normal pattern of venous outflow. At the Stanford Lymphedema Center, we have also become interested in the potential contributory role of venous outflow obstruction in the pathogenesis and responsiveness to complex decongestive therapy of postmastectomy lymphedema. We have attempted to identify the morphologically abnormal patterns through magnetic resonance (MR) imaging of the venous structures in patients with refractory upper extremity lymphedema. In our unpublished observations to date, 40% of such patients have identifiably abnormal venous outflow of the edematous limb. Findings include occlusion of the subclavian or axillary veins as well as frequently observed venous narrowing or kinking along with accentuation of the venous collaterals. These abnormalities on MR imaging of the veins can be substantiated by standard contrast venography. Furthermore, in a small, unpublished patient series, we have observed a substantial therapeutic response of the residual edema in patients subjected to catheter-based, percutaneous venoplasty, with or without stenting of the vein. These results are provocative and certainly warrant further investigation.

Despite major advances in our understanding, much remains to be learned about these conditions. Patients at risk and those with established disease await informed and sophisticated advice from their medical practitioners. For the moment, however, there is a growing body of knowledge surrounding the important precipitating factors in the lymphedema that follows breast carcinoma therapy. Several treatment factors, including the use of radiation and the degree of axillary dissection, significantly impact on the likelihood of lymphedema development. Many additional patient factors, although they often are associated empirically with lymphedema, have no demonstrable relation to the incidence of edema. Patient age, although it is not related specifically to the incidence of postmastectomy lymphedema, seems to influence the likelihood of lymphedema progression, as does the duration of the edema. Hypertension and the prevalence of infection are important comorbidities. Finally, the importance of the multifactorial nature of this edema is stressed. A recognition of the seemingly high incidence of occult venous abnormalities may lead to more widespread application of nonsurgical therapies to reverse edema and, thereby, to an enhanced responsiveness of lymphedema to the conventional, conservative modes of therapy.

REFERENCES

1. Segerstrom K, Bjerle P, Graffman S, Nystrom A. Factors that influence the incidence of brachial oedema after treatment of breast cancer. *Scand J Plast Reconstr Surg Hand Surg* 1992;26:223–7.
2. Schunemann H, Willich N. Secondary lymphedema of the arm following primary therapy of breast carcinoma. *Zentralbl Chir* 1992;117:220–5.
3. Nelson P. Recent advances in treatment of lymphedema of the extremities. *Geratrics* 1966;21:162.
4. Kissin M, Querci della Rovere G, Easton D, Westbury G. Risk of lymphedema following the treatment of breast cancer. *Br J Surg* 1986;73:580–4.
5. Casley-Smith J, Casley-Smith J. Lymphedema initiated by aircraft flights. *Aviat Space Environ Med* 1996;67:52–6.
6. Casley-Smith J. Alterations of untreated lymphedema and its grades over time. *Lymphology* 1995;28:174–85.
7. Pecking A. Treatment of postoperative lymphedema of the upper limb. *Bull Cancer (Paris)* 1991;78:373–7.
8. Halsted WS. The swelling of the arm after operation for cancer of the breast, elephantiasis chirurgica, its causes and prevention. *Bull Johns Hopkins Hosp* 1921;32:309–13.
9. Svensson WE, Mortimer PS, Tohno E, Cosgrove DO. Colour Doppler demonstrates venous flow abnormalities in breast cancer patients with chronic arm swelling. *Eur J Cancer* 1994;30A:657–60.

Psychosocial Aspects of Upper Extremity Lymphedema in Women Treated for Breast Carcinoma

Steven D. Passik, Ph.D.[1]
Margaret V. McDonald, M.S.W.[1,2]

[1] Oncology Symptom Control Research, Community Care, Inc., Indianapolis, Indiana.

[2] Visiting Nurses Association of New York, New York, New York.

BACKGROUND. Lymphedema of the upper extremity following breast carcinoma is highly distressing and disabling.

METHODS. A review is presented of the literature on psychosocial aspects of lymphedema.

RESULTS. Studies have shown that women who develop lymphedema exhibit higher levels of psychological, social, sexual, and functional morbidity than women with breast carcinoma who do not develop this complication. Women who have poor social support, pain, lymphedema in the dominant hand, and/or a passive and avoidant coping style report the highest levels of disability.

CONCLUSIONS. Due to the mobidity of lymphedema once it develops, prevention and information given early are extremely important. However, the recommendations made to women sometimes involve considerable changes in lifestyle but are not based on solid, prospective evidence. In addition, how to best impart and time information about lymphedema pre- and postoperatively require investigation. In this paper, the authors discuss the psychological and functional impact of lymphedema and strategies for intervention and research to help women prevent the condition or enhance coping with it once it develops. *Cancer* 1998;83:2817–20.
© *1998 American Cancer Society.*

KEYWORDS: lymphedema, breast cancer, psychological distress, coping.

Breast carcinoma continues to be the most frequently occurring carcinoma in women. Presently, approximately one in every eight women will develop the disease.[1] Great strides have been made in the treatment of breast carcinoma that have reduced the risk of recurrence and improved survival rates. Thus, as with many other forms of cancer, breast carcinoma is a chronic illness requiring ongoing care and monitoring. With this transformation of the disease into a chronic one comes a greater emphasis on symptom management, quality of life, and the expectation on the part of patients, their families, and caregivers that the patient will attempt to maintain as normal a life style as possible. One problematic condition for women recovering from breast carcinoma surgery or radiation, which, until recently, has received minimal attention, is lymphedema. Although the minority of women develop this condition after treatment, nearly the entire population needs to be informed of the preventative measures necessary to minimize risk. The functional and psychological adjustment needed to accept preventive life style alterations or adhere to treatment regimens requires time and, sometimes, additional supportive intervention.

Lymphedema is an abnormal swelling and collection of excessive tissue protein in the body due to an interruption or obstruction of the lymphatic vessels by a tumor, fibrosis, or inflammation. Women with

Presented at the American Cancer Society Lymphedema Workshop, New York, New York, February 20–22, 1998.

Address for reprints: Steven D. Passik, Ph.D., Community Care, Inc., 115 West 19th Street, Indianapolis, IN 46202.

Received July 2, 1998; accepted August 20, 1998.

breast carcinoma who undergo axillary lymph node dissection or radiation are at risk of scarring and infection, possibly causing blockages in the upper extremity. Reports of the prevalence of upper extremity lymphedema vary widely, ranging from 6.7% to 62.5%.[2-4] These findings are hard to reconcile, because the criteria for defining lymphedema are not standardized, and the various prevalence studies are not consistent in the length of follow-up.[5] There is general agreement that the risk for lymphedema is greatest among women who undergo axillary dissection followed by radiation. The degree of swelling can be mild to severe and can occur immediately in the posttreatment period or several years later. There may be a loss of normal sensation in the affected limb along with skin changes (pitting, abrasions, cellulitis). Untreated, the affected limb can become very large and heavy, and the skin loses its elasticity. In addition, upper extremity lymphedema predisposes women to the development of severe acute or chronic infection.[6]

Psychological and Functional Morbidity Associated with Lymphedema

Problems encountered by women experiencing lymphedema include the disturbing weight of the affected limb and the physical disfigurement of the condition.[5] The heaviness and size of the arm may put substantial limitations on functioning. Women experiencing this condition may have difficulties with performing the tasks needed for their job; they may be unable to complete household responsibilities and, in severe cases, may need assistance with daily care activities. The enlarged size of the arm also may prevent women from wearing their usual clothing. Thus, lymphedema, especially if it is untreated or under-treated, can cause serious disturbances in a patient's quality of life, with additional consequences of psychological distress, depression, social inhibition, and sexuality concerns. Research has demonstrated significant psychological morbidity in patients with lymphedema.[7-9] Tobin and colleagues[7] found that, matched with controls, patients with lymphedema had greater anxiety, depression, adjustment problems, and difficulty in the vocational, domestic, social, and sexual domains. Physical, sexual, and psychological functioning problems also were reported in a study completed by Passik and colleagues.[9] This study listed the presence of pain, lack of social support, avoidant coping, and dominant affected extremity as predictors of greater dysfunction.

Many patients with lymphedema may see the development of this condition as a secondary blow to their physical and emotional well being. They have survived their breast carcinoma in dealing with the initial diagnosis and proceeded through the recommended treatment. The development of lymphedema, whether it is weeks or years after the cancer treatment, can bring back with full force the emotions associated with feeling ill, feeling different from peers, or feeling that "I will never be able to get on with my life." Negative body image perceptions may arise with new concerns about social and sexual interactions. Although the breast carcinoma and procedures to treat it can be quite extensive and can alter body image, the disfigurement is not visible except in intimate situations. Cosmetic surgery, clothing, and prosthetics make is easier to keep the condition private if desired. The visible appearance of lymphedema or of the garments used in its treatment can make privacy issues more difficult, causing social anxieties and constant social reminders of the carcinoma experience. The compression garments themselves are considered unsightly by many women and can lead to decreased social activity. The disfigurement of lymphedema affecting the hand in particular is difficult to conceal, can be painful, and can cause decreased fine motor coordination. Problems in sexuality, common after the treatment for breast carcinoma, may worsen in women experiencing lymphedema. For those feeling unattractive, self-consciousness can hinder intimate relations.

Predictors of Psychological and Functional Morbidity

Not all women who develop lymphedema will have problems adjusting to the challenges posed by living with the condition, but identification of those who are at greater risk for developing psychological problems may improve the outcomes of treatment and management of the condition in many domains, cosmetic and functional. Pain is a complication of lymphedema that causes a great deal of distress and dysfunction for a subset of women, and it is generally somewhat undertreated. When women have painful edema, they may have even greater feelings that things are out of their control and that there is something wrong with their body. Frequently, pain sparks fears of recurrence and intrusive thoughts about cancer.

A lack of social support also has been found to be associated with increased physical interference, psychological distress, and sexual difficulties.[9] Feelings of isolation may heighten the avoidance and social withdrawal associated with lymphedema. Conversely, social contacts can provide assistance with daily activities when needed in severe cases as well as instilling a sense of worth and practical strategies to enhance coping.

In a related study, Passik and colleagues[9] identified an avoidant coping style as another significant predictor of adjustment difficulties for women experiencing lymphedema. Greater psychological morbidity and physical dysfunction as well as an increase in body image concerns were reported by women who relied on passive and avoidant coping methods. Finally, this study also found that women with upper extremity lymphedema in their dominant hand are at greater risk for psychological distress than those women with upper extremity lymphedema in their nondominant limb. The direct impact of greater limitations with an affected dominant limb most likely accounts for this finding.

Interventions for Women with Lymphedema: Prevention and Treatment

Due to the morbidity associated with upper extremity lymphedema once it develops, prevention is an important and natural starting point in the effort to improve quality of life for women with breast carcinoma after surgery and radiation. However, what recommendations to make to women are anything but clear and well studied at this time. Health care professionals are able to provide a few simple recommendations to women postsurgery or postradiation of how they can reduce their risk of developing lymphedema. Avoiding some forms of injury or trauma require only simple strategies that do not necessitate extensive changes in life style. This is not true of other recommendations, however. There are many recommendations (i.e., limit exercise or air travel) that can have a great impact on personal life style (and some recommendations are somewhat conflicting, i.e., reduce weight/blood pressure but limit exercise). It is problematic that none of the recommendations are based on prospective evidence. Simpler suggestions are made to women not to lift heavy objects, or to get blood drawn, or to have blood pressure readings taken from the limb at risk. They should do dishes or gardening wearing gloves because of the exposure to detergents/chemicals and the possibility of cuts. Not cutting cuticles, wearing loose jewelry, and carrying the handbag on the unaffected arm are other common recommendations. It is difficult to advise women to accept major life style changes with limited, research-based evidence that it will provide a benefit. Helping patients overcome the ambiguity and lack of knowledge in this area and helping them make choices about life style and reasonable precautions is a task for the primary treatment team.

Prevention efforts and the imparting of information about lymphedema should begin with presurgical discussion and is a key part of informed consent for surgery and axial node dissection. In these early discussions, the clinician needs to be careful not to overburden the patient with too many fearful thoughts of the consequences of treatment given the high anxiety typical of tis time period. The focus should be on sharing basic information with women about lymphedema. These issues should be revisited in more detail postoperatively, opening up the conversation about how these preventive measures may impact the patient's life style. A positive approach may help women make a behavioral investment and help them feel active in promoting their health postoperatively rather than simply imparting a list of restrictions. Future adherence to prevention programs may be influenced by anxiety and stress that patients may feel about their disease, their treatment, and their overall outlook for prognosis. These issues required prospective study to help understand the optimal timing and manner in which impart this information.

For women who do develop lymphedema, those at risk of experiencing the deleterious emotional effects of the condition should be identified early. Assessment of pain, social functioning, sexual functioning, and social support would comprise an appropriate evaluation. Inquiries into the sexual domain frequently are avoided, although relatively simple questions about premorbid levels of sexual activity and changes due to lymphedema can be used to identify the patients who are in need of formal sex therapy tailored for cancer patients and survivors.[10] Mental health professionals along with members of the treatment team should work to help women adjust and adapt and also to focus on improving compliance with rehabilitative efforts. Lymphedema treatment can be rigorous and and very difficult for women who are depressed, anxious, or in pain. The principle idea of lymphedema therapies is to increase pressure across the affected limb in order to decrease the amount of fluid that is produced and foster removal of excess fluid by any remaining functional lymphatics. This pressure may be applied by using pumps, massage, compression garments, and exercise. Good skin care is essential. These procedures require the commitment and persistence of the patient. The treatment may be time consuming and may require frequent follow-up visits to the clinic. Because the single most important factor in the management of lymphedema is patient compliance,[11,12] the time it takes to assess the patient's adjustment to the condition and the treatment is crucial.

For patients who need more extensive psychological intervention, individual and group therapy modalities that combine cognitive-behavioral, supportive, and insight-oriented techniques along with psychopharmacologic approaches all have a possible role in treating the problems encountered with lymphedema.

The mental health issues can be addressed by bolstering the patient's sense of worth. The disfigurement of the affected limb needs to be put in perspective to the overall well being of the woman and the other positive attributes of her physical self. Cosmetic groups for female carcinoma patients also can assist with discovering ways to diminish the impact of the edema on overall appearance and emphasize a woman's positive qualities. Role playing in which the patient can develop ways of answering questions and dealing with reactions that the patient may encounter in social situations may prove useful. Sexuality concerns also should be addressed. Behavioral techniques are an important aspect of sexual therapy and would best be offered by a therapist with experience in working with carcinoma patients. Although psychiatric disorders in patients with lymphedema are the exception, symptoms should be assessed continually to determine whether a major depression or anxiety disorder is present. If depression develops, then psychopharmacologic interventions can be helpful. Medications need to be chosen with the lymphedema in mind. For example, antidepressants that cause weight gain should be avoided unless those that do not cause weight gain first prove to be ineffective. Establishing a psychoeducational and support group within the clinic may help patients to deal with the lymphedema in a variety of ways. The acceptance of preventative strategies, the adaption of better coping methods, the decreased isolation that often accompanies the condition, and the identification of patients in need of formal consultation are all potential benefits of a support group.[9] With a multidisciplinary approach to this neglected problem, the psychological morbidity associated with lymphedema can be diminished.

REFERENCES

1. Parker SL, Tong T, Bolden S, Wingo PA. Cancer statistics, 1997. *CA Cancer J Clin* 1997;47:5–27.
2. Markowitz J, Wilcox JP, Helm PA. Lymphedema incidence after specific postmastectomy therapy. *Arch Phys Med* 1981; 62:449–52.
3. Larson D, Weinstein M, Goldberg I, et al. Edema of the arm as a function of the extent of axillary surgery in patients with Stage I–II carcinoma of the breast treated with primary radiotherapy. *Int J Radiat Oncol Biol Phys* 1986:1575–82.
4. Kissin MW, Della Rovere GQ, Easton D, Westbury G. Risk of lymphoedema following the treatment of breast cancer. *Br J Surg* 1986;73:580–4.
5. Farncombe M, Daniels G, Cross L. Lymphedema: the seemingly forgotten complication. *J Pain Symp Manage* 1994;9: 269–76.
6. Mortimer PS. Investigation and management of lymphoedema. *Vasc Med Rev* 1990;1:1–20.
7. Tobin M, Lacey HJ, Meyer L, Mortimer PS. The psychological morbidity of breast cancer-related arm swelling. *Cancer* 1993;72:3248–52.
8. Maunsell E, Brisson J, Deschenes L. Arm problems and psychological distress after surgery for breast cancer. *Can J Surg* 1993;36:315–20.
9. Passik SD, Newman M, Brennan M, Tunkel R. Predictors of psychological distress, sexual dysfunction and physical functioning among women with upper extremity lymphedema related to breast cancer. *Psycho-Oncology* 1995;4:255–63.
10. Passik S, Newman M, Brennan M, Holland J. Psychiatric consultation for women undergoing rehabilitation for upper-extremity lymphedema following breast cancer treatment. *J Pain Symptom Manage* 1993;8:226–33.
11. Rose KE, Taylor HM, Twycross RG. Long-term compliance with treatment in obstructive arm lymphedema in cancer. *Palliat Med* 1991:52–5.
12. Zeissler RH, Rose GB, Nelson PA. Postmastectomy lymphedema: late results of treatment in 385 patients. *Arch Phys Med Rehab* 1972;53:159–6.

Overview of Treatment Options and Review of the Current Role and Use of Compression Garments, Intermittent Pumps, and Exercise in the Management of Lymphedema

Michael J. Brennan, M.D.[1]
Linda T. Miller, P.T.[2]

[1] Bridgeport Hospital, Bridgeport, Connecticut.

[2] Breast Cancer Physical Therapy Center, Philadelphia, Pennsylvania.

BACKGROUND. Lymphedema is a relatively frequent complication following the management of breast carcinoma. Numerous therapeutic interventions have been offered to treat this potentially disabling and disfiguring condition. Consensus has not been attained among oncologists, surgeons, psychiatrists, and physical therapists concerning the appropriate treatment of lymphedema.

METHODS. This review provides an overview of those treatment regimens that have been used in the past and, in some instances, have gone on to provide the foundation for the most widely prescribed interventions currently employed for the management of upper extremity lymphedema following breast carcinoma treatment. The use of intermittent pneumatic compression pumps as a part of an integrated multidisciplinary treatment approach incorporating garments, exercises, and massage also is discussed.

RESULTS. A review of available literature suggests that a variety of traditional and commonly available techniques, when used appropriately in a multidisciplinary fashion, may lessen the cosmetic and physical impairments associated with acquired lymphedema. The role of surgery is unclear. Pharmacotherapies are a promising adjunct to manual and mechanical therapies.

CONCLUSIONS. The appropriate use of readily available treatment approaches may lessen the severity of acquired lymphedema following breast carcinoma therapy. A comprehensive therapeutic approach should be employed in the management of lymphedema, including attention to the functional, cosmetic, and emotional sequelae of this potentially disabling condition. To that end, a recommendation for a comprehensive treatment regimen is provided. *Cancer* **1998;83:2821–7.**
© *1998 American Cancer Society.*

KEYWORDS: compression garments, intermittent pumps, exercise, upper extremity lymphedema.

Lymphedema remains an incurable consequence of axillary node surgery and radiation. It has been defined as an abnormal accumulation of tissue proteins, edema, and chronic inflammation within an extremity.[1] Persons afflicted with this condition may have significant associated problems, including pain, impaired extremity function, unsatisfactory cosmesis, and a variety of psychological and social issues.[2–4] Treatment regimens have been prescribed in an effort to mitigate swelling and the protean complications of this condition. Therapeutic efforts remain focused on minimizing the edema and on reversing and restoring the functional and cosmetic nature of the limb. In addition, improved edema control also has been reported as

Presented at the American Cancer Society Lymphedema Workshop, New York, New York, February 20–22, 1998.

Address for reprints: Michael J. Brennan, M.D., 226 Mill Hill Avenue, Bridgeport, CT 06610.

Received July 2, 1998; accepted August 20, 1998.

a means to minimize the risk of chronic and recurrent acute infections of the affected limb.[2]

TREATMENT

The treatment of lymphedema is difficult, multidisciplinary in nature, and, even in the best outcomes, costly and time consuming.[1,5–8] The goal of therapy is to ease the amount of swelling experienced by the patient in order to retain or restore function and cosmesis to the affected limb. It is important to communicate with the patient that multiple modalities and an interdisciplinary approach are needed and that a protracted course of therapy may be required to provide adequate control of swelling.

The quality of the data supporting the varied treatment options purported to be effective in the management of lymphedema is inconsistent. Certain data, specifically, those studies evaluating pump use, at least in some instances, are controlled. However, the majority of reports advocating certain therapeutic options appear to have been obtained by means of uncontrolled, nonrandomized trials or by anecdotal experience. Despite this, a rational assessment of treatment options may permit the prescription of safe and potentially effective interventions.[5]

The therapies available for edema reduction may be divided into three general categories: rehabilitative interventions, pharmacologic therapies, and surgery. Complex decongestive therapies, a multidisciplinary and comprehensive treatment approach incorporating specialized massage, skin care, bandaging, and exercise, will be addressed in a separate section of this supplement.

REHABILITATIVE THERAPIES

There are several common rehabilitative interventions that are used to try to reduce edema. These include elevation, massage, and the application of external pressure. Rehabilitation interventions typically are applied at therapy centers by certified therapists, such as physical and occupational therapists, generally in concert with a prescribing physician. Other individuals, including nurses and licensed massage therapists, may employ these techniques as well. In addition to direct edema reduction, therapists may perform functional assessments and, thus, identify and address issues such as limitations in range of motion, pain, and impaired activities of daily living.

Elevation

Elevation, which typically is not thought of as a form of rehabilitation, is among the first interventions generally recommended by physiatrists, oncologists, and surgeons.[6,7,9] The mechanism of action of elevation in the management of lymphedema is unclear. It has been suggested that elevation of an extremity reduces intravascular hydrostatic pressure, thereby decreasing those intravascular forces responsible in part for production of lymph.[8,10]

There are no data on the efficacy of elevation in the treatment of lymphedema. Recommended guidelines are not available, and most clinicians appear to base their continued prescription of elevation on personal or anecdotal experience. Compliance with elevation is untenable: Continuous elevation during the course of the day can impede the function of the individual perhaps more severely than the edema itself. Efforts may be made to elevate the affected limb at night during sleep; however, clinical experience suggests that this is virtually impossible and inevitably will fail. Therefore, elevation may be warranted as an adjunct to therapies, but it is not to be considered a mainstay of edema therapies.

Massage Therapies

Traditional massage techniques, including self-administered retrograde massage, are prescribed routinely as part of a multidisciplinary treatment approach to lymphedema.[1,2,5,9,11] Effleurage, a classical form of massage, retrograde self-massage, and stroking may produce a mild pressure gradient, acting to remove edema from the limb. They also may stimulate inherent mechanisms within the limb to aid in the removal of lymphatic fluid. These traditional techniques may be administered by a certified therapist, by the spouse of a patient, or by the patient themselves after proper instruction.

Vodder developed manual lymphatic drainage as a specific technique for the treatment of lymphedema.[12] Manual lymphatic drainage has been reported to be effective when used in combination with other antiedema efforts, such as complex decongestive therapies, as well as in combination with an intermittent compression pump and complex decongestive therapies. Manual lymphatic drainage is a specialized, distinct form of massage, incorporating regional massage as well as treatment of the affected limb.

Exercise

Exercise is an integral component of virtually all rehabilitation. The role of exercise in the management of upper extremity lymphedema is not well defined. Data supporting exercise programs are lacking. Specifically, the type, intensity, frequency, and under what conditions exercise may be employed safely to reduce swelling have not been defined fully.

Data support the benefits of exercise in enhancing lymph flow[13,14] as well as improving protein resorbtion,[15] both of which are integral in lymphedema management. Lymph flow occurs as a result of inspiratory reduction in the intrathoracic pressure associated with inspiration,[16] leading to speculation that increased pulmonary work associated with various forms of exercise may assist in the management of swelling. It has also been found that compromise in upper extremity venous drainage is noted frequently in individuals with lymphedema.[17] It has therefore been suggested that flexibility training may lessen the role that soft tissue contracture might play in impeding blood and lymphatic drainage.

Clinical experience suggests and it has been reported that combinations of flexibility, aerobic training, and strengthening in combination with the use of compression wrapping, manual lymphatic drainage, and compression pumps have produced significant benefits in women with lymphedema.[18] In addition, such a program also enhances the overall level of function of the extremity and the patient.[19,20]

All exercise regimens require individualization. Proper assessment of flexability, strength, and aerobic capacity should be performed prior to instituting treatment.[21] Gradual progression of exercises, both aerobic and strengthening, should be expected. However, frequent reassessment of the extremity is mandated to assure that worsening edema does not develop. All resistance and aerobic exercises should be done when the patient either is wrapped appropriately or is wearing a well-fitting compression garment.

Contraindications to exercises are few. Cardiac and pulmonary disease should be considered relative contraindications. Complications include muscle pain and, occasionally, worsening of edema. Patients should be counseled concerning both of these prior to instituting any treatment program.

External Compression

External compression is defined as the application of any external pressure to the limb. External compression in the management of edema is used for two reasons: to try to reduce edema formation and to aid in the removal of excess lymph fluid already accumulated within the limb. Compression may be realized through a variety of techniques and technologies.

Compression garments

Compression garments are used widely in the management of lymphedema. Garments are available in both custom-made and prefabricated varieties. Also, garments may be obtained in a gradient format in which distal compression is greater than proximal compression.[22] In addition, sleeves have been intro-

duced recently that permit manual, inflatable pressures against the limb.

There are data supporting the use of garments in the management of lymphedema.[22,23] The mechanism of action of garments remains unclear. It is likely that garments aid in reducing swelling by lessening the amount of edema formed within the involved extremity. It remains unclear whether garments actually reduce the existing edema within the limb. In addition, garments lend a measure of protection against external incidental trauma, such as burns and lacerations. They also may protect against intrinsic trauma to the limb that occurs as a result of chronically increased interstitial pressures.[1] It has been suggested that this increased pressure is exerted against the skin and other subcutaneous tissues that aid in maintaining interstitial fluid homeostasis.[1,2,8,12,24] These tissues ultimately will stretch as a result of this relentless force. Use of a garment or other type of wrap, such as a bandage, likely relieves the skin and subcutaneous tissues from bearing this increased pressure. This shift of pressure bearing from the skin to the garment protects these tissues from eventual stretching.

Selection of garment type and recommended guidelines for their use remain unclear. Choice of particular garments likely occurs based on clinical experience. There are no data supporting the preferential selection of either prefabricated or customized garments. Cost and patient tolerance to the garment warrant consideration when prescribing. Prefabricated garments usually are less expensive than customized garments. The use of a glove or gauntlet depends on whether the hand is involved. Hand swelling may develop or become problematic by the use of an arm sleeve. Patients should be made aware of this potential complication prior to instituting the use of a garment. Consideration should be given to either a long wrist piece gauntlet or a one-piece, customized sleeve if hand swelling persists. Customized garments may be needed for those patients who are difficult to fit or those in need of some assistive device to facilitate donning or removal. Garments typically last no more than 3–6 months: They should be replaced when they begin to lose their elasticity.

Recommended parameters for the use and prescription of garments vary. Pressures ranging from 30 mm Hg to 60 mm Hg are prescribed routinely. Garment use for 20 hours per day and longer has been suggested.[1,5,11,12,24,25] Bertelli et al.[23] have reported statistically significant reduction of edema in patients who wore garments for 6 consecutive hours per day. A multivariate analysis noted superior reduction in those women who had not had significant weight gain following treatment for breast carcinoma. Using garments during physical activity and exercise has been advocated.[11,12]

Compliance is difficult for patients, because even the most customized garment typically is uncomfortable, unsightly, and laborious to put on. Patient education may improve compliance with the prescribed garment.

Contraindications to the use of compression garments are few. Insensate extremities need to be inspected often to ensure skin integrity. Infections within the limb may make the use of garments more difficult because of pain. Open wounds should not be considered a contraindication. Complications from the use of compression garments include inducing or worsening hand swelling. Skin irritation may occur from contact dermatitis.

Pneumatic compression

The prescription and use of intermittent pneumatic pumps has been the mainstay of lymphedema therapy in the United States for many years. It continues to be a reimbursed therapy for lymphedema by federal and third-party payers. Several controlled studies have documented their usefulness in the treatment of this condition, thereby supporting their continued use.[26–31] Despite this, several important issues, such as optimum pumping pressures, the length and frequency of pumping sessions, and the need for continuation of pumping after initial reduction has been attained, have yet to be determined. In addition, misuse and the inappropriate prescription of these devices by clinicians untrained in the selection, parameters, and effective protocols has led to a perception among many practitioners and patients that pumps are ineffective.

A variety of pumps are available. They range in cost from several hundred dollars for simpler devices to several thousand dollars for more advanced units. Pumps may be single chambered or may come with several compartments. Multiple-chamber pumps typically inflate from distal to proximal, thereby producing a wave of pressure that ascends the extremity, theoretically bringing edema fluid with it. It has been suggested that this allows the retained fluid to be brought to functional lymphatics that might aid in its removal.

Guidelines for pump selection and their use are unclear. No individual pump appears to have a distinct advantage or to be inherently superior over any other.[5,8] Likewise, patients have a wide variety of responses and tolerances to these devices. Studies assessing efficacy of certain pumps have been reported. Unfortunately, no comparative studies assessing the relative efficacy of pumps are available. One study has found that a multichambered device was effective in a small population of patients who had not responded previously to a single-chamber device.[27] However, another study noted superior reduction of swelling from a single-chamber device compared with a device with multiple chambers.[31] It has therefore been recommended that a trial comparing pumping devices be made before a unit is obtained for patients to use at home.[5]

Initial pumping sessions may be performed in either inpatient or outpatient settings.[5,7,29] Optimal pressure ranges, inflation/deflation cycles, and the length and frequency of individual pumping sessions have not been established. In a nonrandomized study, statistically significant reduction in edema was described with a sequential gradient pump when administered over a 48-hour period. Several authors have suggested determining pumping pressures by calculating the mean arterial pressure.[27,28] Others have recommended pressures ranging from 80 mm Hg to 110 mm Hg pumping 4–8 hours per day.[29] Yamakazi et al. recommended pressure settings at or near 80 mm Hg.[32] Long term responses to a combination of pumping and garments have been reported, including at least partial maintenance of reduction in edema in 36 of 49 patients who were treated for lower extremity edema for a mean of 25 months.[29]

It has been purported that pumps may be ineffective and perhaps dangerous.[2,12,33] However, extensive clinical experience does not support these claims. Pumps used at relatively low pressures also have been advocated as part of a comprehensive program including manual lymph drainage, bandaging, and exercise.

Complications from pumping therapy are few. Entrapment neuropathies may become symptomatic during the course of pumping. Pain may limit the maximum pressure employed. Contraindications include infection in the limb, local or proximate malignancy, anticoagulated patients, and deep vein thrombosis. Use of palliative pumping has been described in patients with advanced carcinoma to restore function and as an adjunct to pain control.[5]

SURGICAL THERAPY

Surgical therapy for the management of lymphedema may be divided into two general categories: debulking or reduction surgery, in which the limb has excess fluid and tissues removed, and functional or physiologic surgery, in which efforts to enhance lymphatic function are undertaken. The Charles procedure, first described in 1912, is a debulking procedure. Although variations of this procedure are still performed,[34] significant drawbacks, including poor wound healing and infection, have been associated with it.[35,36] Case reports suggesting suction lipectomy as a means of reducing the size of an involved extremity in patients who have failed less aggressive interventions have been published.[37–39] Long term follow-up is not available for these cases. It also has been suggested that a combination of reduction surgery and conservative interventions should be considered for certain severe cases.[40]

A variety of surgical techniques have been described that are purported to enhance lymph removal from an edematous extremity. These functional or physiologic surgical procedures include lymphangioplasty,[41] omental and pedicle flaps,[35,36] and myocutaneous flaps.[42] The microlymphatic-venous anastomosis (LVA) consists of grafts between lymphatic vessels or nodes and proximate venous systems to allow removal of lymph.[41] Several studies of involved upper extremities found good relief in 50–77% of patients treated with LVA.[41,43–49] However, the number of patients studied suffering from postbreast carcinoma therapy lymphedema was small in all of these studies. Another limitation is that recurrence of swelling to some degree was reported to have occurred in most patients undergoing this procedure.[44] O'Brien et al. have reported superior reduction in patients treated with the combined technique incorporating LVA with a reduction procedure versus those treated with LVA alone.[45]

DRUG THERAPY

Pharmacotherapy has been suggested as an adjunct to the treatment of lymphedema. Coumarin, a benzopyrone, reportedly has a beneficial effect on lymphedema. This class of drug may work by stimulating proteolysis by macrophages as well as increasing the absolute number of macrophages within the edematous extremity.[50] Two randomized, placebo-controlled, cross-over studies found statistically significant benefits in patients with lymphedema who received benzopyrones for several months.[50,51] Unfortunately, there are no data about the long term effects or potential toxicities of these agents.

Other drugs have been used routinely in the treatment of lymphedema and associated infection. No controlled data exist that support the treatment of all patients with acquired lymphedema with antibiotics. Use of antibiotics is appropriate in the treatment of acute and chronic infections, such as cellulitis and lymphangitis. Selection of antibiotics and adequate treatment course has not been elucidated. There are no data supporting the use of diuretics for long term management of this type of swelling. Some authors

suggest that use of these agents may be deleterious, although these claims are unsubstantiated.[9]

TREATMENT RECOMMENDATIONS

A rationale for a comprehensive treatment regimen may be devised from a review of those treatments available and by their cogent application in an interdisciplinary model. Physical, psychological, and functional assessment must precede the institution of any course of therapy. Likewise, comprehensive treatment by a multidisciplinary team should be employed to best meet the complex physical, functional, and emotional needs of these patients.

The daily use of compression garments, whether prefabricated or customized, together with intermittent pneumatic compression pumps has realized reasonable compliance and success. These interventions may be used to form the core of a lymphedema management program. Individualized and tailored pumping programs for patients cannot be intuited; therefore, they require an empiric basis for each woman deemed appropriate. Pump selection should be based on measurable efficacy and tolerability, as evidenced by serial assessment with each patient. After determining which device should be prescribed, thorough education in the pump's limitations and use must be undertaken to best assure continued compliance. Ongoing reassessment of the efficacy and tolerance of individual components of the treatment program should be made prior to any final determination of a home maintenance program. Exercise focusing on improving flexability, strength, and aerobic capacity will function both to enhance lymphatic removal and to aid the patient in returning to their highest functional level. Exercise needs to be individualized to meet the specific needs of the patient and to assure safe implementation of such a program. Exercise should be done while wearing a compressive dressing, either bandaging or a well-fit garment. Retrograde massage also should be part of the daily care plan. Medical comorbidities, such as infection and skin breakdown, should be addressed appropriately. Psychiatric and/or psychological therapies and referral should be instituted as needed.

CONCLUSIONS

There is no cure for acquired lymphedema, but treatment options are available for controlling swelling. Unfortunately, the evidence supporting many of these forms of treatment is less than optimal. A multidimensional approach to care provided in an interdisciplinary team, including garments, massage, exercise, and the appropriate use of sequential pumps at a sufficient pressure, form the core program for most patients with lymphedema. Surgery is best reserved for those individuals in whom conservative care has been ineffective. Surveillance for infection and other complications, including psychological distress, should be maintained after a patient has been placed on a home program.

REFERENCES

1. Grabois M. Breast cancer. Postmastectomy lymphedema. State of the art review. *Phys Med Rehabil Rev* 1994;8:267–77.
2. Foldi E, Foldi M, Clodius L. The lymphedema chaos: a lancet. *Ann Plast Surg* 1989;22:505–15.
3. Passik S, Newmann M, Brennan M, Holland J. Psychiatric consultation for women undergoing rehabilitation for upper-extremity lymphedema following breast cancer treatment. *J Pain Sympt Manage* 1993;8(4):226–33.
4. Passik S, Newmann M, Brennan M, Tunkel R. Predictors of psychiatric distress in patients with upper extremity lymphedema. *Psycho-Oncology* 1995;4:255–63.
5. Brennan MJ. Lymphedema following the surgical treatment of breast cancer: a review of pathophysiology and treatment. *J Pain Symp Manage* 1992;7(2):110–6.
6. Levinson SF. Rehabilitation of the patient with cancer or human immunodeficiency virus. Rehabilitation medicine principles and practice. 2nd ed. Dellisa JA, editor. Philadelphia: JB Lippincott, 1993:916–33.
7. Nelson PA. Rehabilitation of patients with lymphedema. In: Krusen's hand book of physical medicine and rehabilitation. 4th ed. Kottke FJ, Lehmann JF, editors. Philadelphia: Saunders 1990:1134–9.
8. Brennan MJ, Depompolo RW, Garden FH. Focused review: postmastectomy lymphedema. *Arch Phys Med Rehabil* 1996; 77:S74–80.
9. Garden FH, Gillis TA. Principles of cancer rehabilitation. In: Physical medicine and rehabilitation. Braddon RL, editor. Philadelphia: Saunders, 1996:1199–214.
10. Guyton AC. Human physiology and mechanisms of disease. 5th ed. Philadelphia: WB Saunders Co., 1992:202–3.
11. Foldi E, Foldi M, Weissleder H. Conservative treatment of lymphoedema of the limbs. *Angiology* 1985;36(3):171–80.
12. Casley-Smith JR, Casley-Smith JR. Modern treatment of lymphedema I complex physical therapy: the first 200 Australian limbs. *Aust J Dermatol* 1992;33(2):61–8.
13. Motimer PS. Managing lymphoedema. *Clin Exp Dermatol* 1995;20:98–106.
14. Motimer PS. Investigation and management of lymphoedema. *Vasc Med Rev* 1990;1:1–20.
15. LeDuc O, Bourgeois A, et al. Bandages: scintigraphic demonstration of its efficacy on colloidal protein reabsorption during muscle activity. In: Congress Book XII. International Congress of Lymphology, 1989:421–3.
16. Whittlinger H. Textbook of Dr. Vodder's manual of lymphatic drainage, I. Heidelberg, Germany: Karl R. Haug Publishers, 1982;64.
17. Svensson WE, Mortimer PS, et al. Colour Doppler demonstrates venous flow abnormalities in breast cancer patients with chronic arm swelling. *Eur J Cancer* 1994;30A(5):657–60.
18. Miller LT. Lymphedema: unlocking the doors to successful treatment. *Innov Oncol Nurs* 1994;10:58–62.
19. Winningham M, Nail L, et al. Fatigue and the cancer experience: the state of the knowledge." *Oncol Nurs Forum* 1994; 21:23–36.
20. MacVicar MG, Winningham M, et al. Effects of aerobic interval training on cancer patients' functional capacity. *Nurs Res* 1989;38:348–51.
21. American College of Sports Medicine. Guidelines for exercise testing and prescription. Philadelphia: Lea and Febiger, 1991:179.
22. Johnson G, Kupper C, Farrar DJ, Swallow RT. Graded compression stockings. *Arch Surg* 1982;117:69–72.
23. Bertelli G, Venturini M, Forno G, Macchiavello F, Dini D. An analysis of prognostic factors in response to conservative treatment of postmastectomy lymphedema. *Surg Gynecol Obstet* 1992;175(5):455–60.
24. Casley-Smith JR. Modern treatment of lymphedema. *Mod Med Aust* 1992:70–83.
25. Ohkuma M. Lymphedema treated by microwave and elastic dressing. *Int J Dermatol* 1992;31(9):660–3.
26. Bunce IH, Mirolo BR, Hennessy JM, Ward LC, Jones LC. Post-mastectomy lymphoedema treatment and measurement. *Med J Aust* 1994;161(2):125–8.
27. Klein MJ, Alexander MA, Wright JM, Redmond CK, LaGasse AA. Treatment of adult lower extremity lymphedema with the Wright Linear pump: statistical analysis of a clinical trial. *Arch PM&R* 1988;69:202–6.
28. Kim-Sing C, Basco VE. Postmastectomy lymphedema treated with the Wright linear pump. *Can J Surg* 1987;5:368–70.
29. Pappas CJ, O'Donnell TF Jr. Long-term results of compression treatment for lymphedema. *J Vasc Surg* 1992;16(4):555–62.
30. Richmand DM, O'Donnell TR Jr, Zelikovski A. Sequential pneumatic compression for lymphedema. A controlled trial. *Arch Surg* 1985;120(10):1116–9.
31. Zanolla R, Monzeglio C, Balzarini A, Martino G. Evaluation of the results of three different methods of postmastectomy lymphedema treatment. *J Surg Oncol* 1984;26(3):210–3.
32. Yamazaki Z, Idezuki Y, Nemoto T, Togawa T. Clinical experiences using pneumatic massage therapy for edematous limbs over the last 10 years. *Angiology* 1988;39(2):154–63.
33. Boris M, Weindorf S, Lasinski B, Boris G. Lymphedema reduction by noninvasive complex lymphedema therapy. *Oncology* 1994;9:95–106.
34. Miller TA. Surgical approach to lymphedema of the arm after mastectomy. *Am J Surg* 1984;148(1):152–6.
35. Savage RC. The surgical management of lymphedema [review]. *Surg Gynecol Obstet* 1985;160(3):283–90.
36. Savage RC. The surgical management of lymphedema [review]. *Surg Gynecol Obstet* 1984;159(5):501–8.
37. Nava VM, Lawrence WT. Liposuction on a lymphedematous arm. *Ann Plast Surg* 1988;21(4):366–8.
38. Sando WC, Nahai F. Suction lipectomy in the management of limb lymphedema. *Clin Plast Surg* 1989;16(2):369–73.
39. Louton RB, Terranova WA. The use of suction curettage as adjunct to the management of lymphedema. *Ann Plast Surg* 1989;22(4):354–7.
40. Zelikovski A, Haddad M, Reiss R. Non-operative therapy combined with limited surgery in management of peripheral lymphedema. *Lymphology* 1986;19(3):106–8.
41. Degni M. Surgical management of selected patients with lymphedema of the extremities. *J Cardiovasc Surg* 1984; 25(6):481–8.
42. Kambayashi J, Ohshiro T, Mori T. Appraisal of myocutaneous flapping for treatment of postmastectomy lymphedema. Case report. *Acta Chir Scand* 1990;156(2):175–7.

43. Filippetti M, Santoro E, Graziano F, Petric M, Rinaldi G. Modern therapeutic approaches to postmastectomy brachial lymphedema. *Microsurgery* 1994;5(8):504–10.

44. Gloviczki P, Fisher J, Hollier L, Pairoler PC, Schirger A, Wahner HW. Microsurgical lymphovenous anastomosis for treatment of lymphedema: a critical review. *J Vasc Surg* 1988;7(5):647–52.

45. O'Brien BM, Mellow CG, Khazanchi RK, Dvir E, Kumar V, Pederson WC. Long-term results after microlymphaticovenous anastomoses for the treatment of obstructive lymphedema. *Plast Reconstruct Surg* 1990;85(4):562–72.

46. Haddad M, Matz E, Zelikovski A, Melloul M, Reiss R. Surgical treatment of limb lymphedema. *Int J Surg* 1988; 73(2):116–8.

47. Ho LC, Lai MF, Yeates M, Fernandez V. Microlymphatic bypass in obstructive lymphoedema. *Br J Plast Surg* 1988; 41(5):475–84.

48. Huang GK, Ju RQ, Liu ZZ. Microlymphaticovenous anastomosis for lymphedema of the breast. *Microsurgery* 1985;6(1): 32–5.

49. Liu XY, Ge BF. Lymphatic venous shunt in the treatment of postmastectomy lymphedema. *Chinese Med J* 1985;98(1): 65–6.

50. Piller NV, Morgan RG, Casley-Smith Jr. A double-blind, cross-over trial of 0-(beta-hydroxyethyl)-rutosides (benzopyrones) in the treatment of lymphoedema of the arms and legs. *Br J Plast Surg* 1988;41(1):20–7.

51. Casley-Smith JR, Morgan RG, Piller NB. Treatment of lymphedema of the arms and legs with 5,6-benzo-[alpha]-pyrone. *N Engl J Med* 1993;329(16):1158–63.

American Cancer Society Lymphedema Workshop

Supplement to **Cancer**

Conservative Approaches to Lymphedema Treatment

Margaret E. Rinehart-Ayres, Ph.D., P.T.

Thomas Jefferson University, College of Health Professions, Philadelphia, Pennsylvania.

BACKGROUND. Upper extremity lymphedema can develop after surgery for breast carcinoma. Once developed, it becomes a chronic problem that women must cope with for the rest of their lives. Steps to prevent lymphedema should begin immediately after surgery. However, there is little information available about what actually causes lymphedema; therefore, it is difficult to prevent, and there is some controversy over how women should be treated once lymphedema has developed.

METHODS. The literature was reviewed to understand the education about arm care provided to women during and after the short hospital stay for breast carcinoma surgery. Evaluation and treatment options for lymphedema and complications resulting from lymphedema were explored.

RESULTS. Women are provided with basic arm care information after surgery; however, many women require reinforcement from health professionals, such as physical or occupational therapists, to reach optimum functional outcomes. If lymphedema does develop, then there are two treatment regimes that have been used. The compression pump, along with skin care, exercise, and compression garments, is one option. However, there is little consistency with the length of time the pump should be used or the optimum number of days required to receive the best results. The second treatment option is known as complex decongestive physiotherapy or complex physical therapy. Arm care, therapeutic exercises, manual lymph drainage, and compression bandages and/or garments comprise this treatment regime. Decreases in lymphedema are noted if women are compliant with the prescribed treatment program.

CONCLUSIONS. Women must be educated about possible complications after breast surgery. This should be a team effort, with physicians, nurses, physical and occupational therapists, and Reach to Recovery volunteers from the American Cancer Society all participating in the process. If women do develop lymphedema, then an individual treatment program must be established, and adherence to the program must be stressed. More research is needed to determine the optimum treatment regime for women who develop lymphedema. *Cancer* **1998;83:2828–32.**
© 1998 American Cancer Society.

KEYWORDS: lymphedema, evaluation, measurement, treatment, Reach to Recovery, prevention, complex decongestive therapy, complex physical therapy, compression pumps, research.

Presented at the American Cancer Society Lymphedema Workshop, New York, New York, February 20–22, 1998.

Address for reprints: Margaret E. Rinehart-Ayres, Ph.D., P.T., Assistant Professor, Thomas Jefferson University, College of Health Professions, 130 South 9th Street, Suite 830 Edison Building, Philadelphia, PA 19107.

Received July 2, 1998; accepted August 20, 1998.

Conventional Approaches to Lymphedema Treatment

I have been charged with the task of exploring the conventional approaches used for the treatment of lymphedema that occurs after surgery for breast carcinoma. This is known as secondary lymphedema, because it usually occurs after a surgical intervention and/or radiation therapy that may damage the lymphatic system. When the delicately balanced lymphatic system is damaged, it may be unable transport fluid, because there is a build-up of protein that attracts fluid and results in a build-up of lymph fluid in the subcutaneous tissues. The excess fluid causes edema, which also predisposes the individual to infection.[1]

There are surgical and nonsurgical interventions. The nonsurgical interventions that are used to treat lymphedema will be presented here, because early treatment usually does not require surgical intervention. Surgical interventions are discussed elsewhere[2–4] in greater detail.

Lymphedema has been identified as a sequelae of surgery by numerous authors.[5–7] It can occur after a radical mastectomy, modified radical mastectomy, segmental mastectomy with axillary dissection, and/or radiation therapy to the chest or axillary area. It is still unclear why some women are more prone to develop lymphedema than others, but it is a significant problem. The incidence of lymphedema has been cited to range from 6% to 62%[8]; however, because women are not monitored routinely for the development of lymphedema after surgery, it is difficult to ascertain the actual figures. Hopefully, with Dr. Petrek's study from Memorial Sloan-Kettering and increased awareness about lymphedema, greater accuracy in reporting will found.

The Hospital Stay

The conventional approach to lymphedema begins with the admission to the hospital for a surgical procedure to treat the breast carcinoma. In the United States, women who have a modified radical mastectomy with axillary dissection usually are admitted to the hospital for 1–2 days. If they choose to have immediate breast reconstruction, then they may be in the hospital for as many as 3–4 days. For the women who choose a segmental mastectomy with axillary sampling, the length of hospitalization may be 1 day, or, in some cases, it may be performed as outpatient surgery. This means that there is very little time for patient education to occur, and, although some hospitals are providing preoperative education, it is not the norm at this time. When women are in the hospital, a sign typically is placed over their bed to remind other health professionals not to perform a venepuncture or to take blood pressure in the involved arm. Some hospitals also are using a pink hospital arm band (developed by Diane Nannery) to help reinforce this issue. This is the first step toward prevention of lymphedema; however, many women are not made aware that this is a life-long recommendation. Women also should be educated that they may need to reinforce lymphedema prevention strategies with their health professionals after discharge.

Women also may be advised to keep their arm elevated and to squeeze a foam ball to help decrease postoperative edema. This is not an activity that

TABLE 1
Arm Care Recommendations

1.	Clean cuts, scratches, pin pricks, hang nails, insect bites, or burns and put antibiotic cream on them
2.	Have injections, venepuncture, and blood pressure done on uninvolved arm
3.	Wear a mitt when reaching into a hot oven
4.	Carry a purse in the opposite arm
5.	Use hand cream to prevent chapping of hand
6.	Wear gloves when washing dishes or gardening or when using strong detergents

women should be encouraged to do routinely after discharge, because it does not prevent lymphedema, and more "normal" movement of the upper extremity is encouraged. Most women are provided with written instructions about incision care, exercises to increase shoulder motion, and activity level after discharge, although written information alone does not seem to be enough. Women may need more one-on-one intervention to understand exactly what types of exercises they should do. There may be information included about arm care (see Table 1), but the need for life-long attention to these issues and strategies of how to compensate for these activities is not stressed. In many cases, the issue of lymphedema is not a high priority for women who have just undergone surgery or for the health professionals that work with them. Recently, in a conversation with a breast surgeon about lymphedema, I was told that she did not talk about lymphedema with her patients right after surgery because she did not want to "frighten them."

During the hospital stay or upon discharge, women can be referred by their doctor or they refer themselves to the American Cancer Society's Reach to Recovery (RTR) program. Many women also are starting to take advantage of another aspect of the RTR program, which is the Early Support program offered to women prior to surgery. It is a peer-modeling program that attempts to match a woman who is contemplating surgery or has undergone surgery for breast carcinoma with a trained RTR visitor who has had similar surgery.[9,10] The trained visitor provides emotional support, answers questions, and reinforces the need to care for the arm after surgery; however, the issue of lymphedema is not always stressed.

In the past, women were most often seen in the hospital; however, because women are discharged within 1 or 2 days after surgery, many visits take place at alternate sites. Women may be visited in their home, a doctor's office, or a coffee shop. Women find these visits to be very beneficial, and physicians and therapists should encourage women to take advantage of this free service.

With the advent of managed care in the American health system, hospital stays are very short. Therefore, referral to physical or occupational therapy is not always a routine activity. It is not typical for women to be referred for rehabilitation for educational purposes or to screen for arm edema as therapists are trained to do. Women often are referred for therapy only after discharge from the hospital, and it is usually because of a limitation in shoulder range of motion or function, although it has been shown that therapeutic intervention can be beneficial to to many women.[11–14]

When Does the Diagnosis of Lymphedema Occur?

Unfortunately, as we have heard earlier in this program, making a diagnosis of lymphedema is not always easy. Some of the barriers to the diagnosis may include that women may not have been educated or may not retain information about the possible development of lymphedema after surgery, that they may not understand the impact that lymphedema may have on their lives or how to detect lymphedema, and that when edema is noted by women, doctors may trivialize the necessity for treatment and may not refer women for early treatment. This means that treatment is delayed, and women may develop a more severe lymphedema because of it.

Lymphedema can occur anytime from a few months to years after surgery.[11,15] If it occurs within a few months of surgery, then it may be identified by the surgeon, medical oncologist, or radiation oncologist. If it occurs years later, then the individual woman may be the first person to observe the edema. She may note that the arm feels heavy, there may be pain and paresthesias, or range of motion and function may be impaired.[16,17] That is why it is imperative that appropriate patient education occurs at the time of surgical treatment. Women should be provided with problem-solving strategies for all aspects of their lives, including home management, return to work outside the home, and exercise and recreational activities. Women may need to make some modifications in how they carry out everyday activities, but they need physical or occupational therapists to help them. Women also should be provided with education regarding how to recognize the onset of lymphedema, what to do if lymphedema develops, and long term implications. If women are educated about this, then some of the long term problems that have been discussed can be prevented.

Treatment Regime

Women who require treatment for lymphedema usually are evaluated by a physician prior to treatment to determine what factors may have contributed to the development of lymphedema. If an infection is present, then antibiotics usually are prescribed. Once the infection has been cured, more aggressive therapeutic intervention can begin.

It is not always easy for physicians or for the women with lymphedema to find a clinic that can offer therapeutic treatment for lymphedema. At the present time, there are not enough centers available or clinicians trained in the management of more severe lymphedema to provide a comprehensive treatment program for women. The National Lymphedema Network and the American Cancer Society are two organizations that can assist women with finding treatment centers.

The initial therapeutic intervention is an evaluation to measure the amount of lymphedema and any other limitations that may be present. Health professionals stress the need to monitor the circumference of the arm, but there is also a need to evaluate the functional activities that are impaired and the impact on societal roles. It is also the time to explain the consequences of lymphedema to the patient and remind them about good arm care. When lymphedema is identified, there are two methods that are used to measure lymphedema. A tape measure is used to measure arm girth or circumference, or a volumeter[18] is used to measure the volume of the arm. It appears that more clinicians are using arm circumference to calculate the volume by using equation for a truncated cone[19] rather than the volumeter. When the volumeter is used, measurements cannot be performed quickly, because it has to be cleaned and sterilized between each use. However, when arm girth is used, there is little consistency among clinicians in the use of landmarks or the distance between measurements, which makes it difficult to compare the results or outcomes between studies or treatment clinics.[5,20,21] The professionals who treat patients with lymphedema should agree on the landmarks and the distance between measurements, such as 10 cm, that should be used. This will help to develop a more consistent approach to evaluation.

When the evaluation is completed, the treatment intervention can begin. There are two types of treatment programs. One method of treatment uses a program of skin care followed by the use of an intermittent sequential compression pump and general upper extremity exercises. The pump has been used for a varied number of days and length of time. Some patients are treated for a single 6–8 hour session,[23] and others are treated for 2–3 hours daily for 3 weeks,[16] so there is little consistency in treatment regimes using pumps. Both regimes encourage women to use an elastic compression sleeve after pumping. There have been varied results in the reduction of lymphedema with the pumps,[2,23] but there is not always regular follow-up to determine whether the reduction is maintained for greater than 6–12 months. This is an important issue because lymphedema is a life-long problem. More research is needed to determine the value of pumps in the treatment of lymphedema.

The second type of treatment program has been gaining more followers each year because of the benefits realized from the treatment. This is known as complex decongestive physiotherapy (CDP) by Földi,[24] who pioneered this approach, or complex physical therapy (CPT) by the Casley-Smiths.[7] This method includes skin care, gentle massage known as manual lymph drainage, and the use of low-stretch compression bandages followed by measurement and prescription of a fitted compression garment when the edema has plateaued. Therapeutic exercises that are included in the program are performed when the garment or bandages are in place. It has been recommended that patients receive treatment 5 days a week for 4 weeks, although this is starting to be questioned by clinicians. Morgan et al.[25] found that the greatest reduction in lymphedema occurred within the first 10 days of treatment, and Boris et al.[26] found that reduction can be maintained up to 3 years if patients are compliant with wearing their compression garments. Thus, there is more research to be done in this area.

Both methods described require that the patient be an active participant in her treatment. She must make a commitment to continue to perform the exercises and skin care as well as wear the compression garment to help control this chronic problem. The compression garments must be replaced every 2–6 months to maintain the proper amount of compression, because they become loose and stretched over a period of time.

It appears that CDP/CPT may be the method of choice for treatment, and more clinicians should be educated about the value of the methods included in this treatment regime. However, more research is required to determine the number of days intensive treatment is necessary for women to receive the optimum benefit. There are at least two reasons to study this issue. The first is because the 4-week intensive program is difficult for women to fit into their busy life style, there are few clinics in the United States that offer this type of program, and there is evidence that the most benefit may occur within the first 10 days of treatment.[25] The second reason is especially important, because the American health system typically does not support such lengthy treatment regimes.

There is pressure from third-party payers to shorten the number of visits required for medical interventions, which in turn, will decrease the cost of care, as demonstrated by the decreased length of hospitals stays for most medical and surgical interventions. We need to determine how to provide optimum care that provides the desired outcomes while maintaining fiscal responsibility.

REFERENCES

1. Mortimer P. Managing lymphoedema. *Clin Exp Dermatol* 1995;20:98–106.
2. Lerner R, Requena R. Upper extremity lymphedema secondary to mammary cancer treatment. *Am J Clin Oncol* 1986; 9(6):481–7.
3. Servelle M. Surgical treatment of lymphedema: a report on 652 cases. *Surg* 1987;101(4):485–95.
4. Morgan RG. Surgery and microsurgery for lymphedema. In: Lymphedema. Casley-Smith JR, Casley-Smith JR, (editors). Adelaide, Australia: The Lymphedema Association of Australia, 1991:176–7.
5. Penzer RD, Patterson MP, Hill LR, Lipsett JA, Desai KR, Vora N, et al. Arm lymphedema in patients treated conservatively for breast cancer: relationship to patient age and axillary node dissection technique. *Int J Radiat Oncol Biol Phys* 1986;12:2079–83.
6. Hardy JR, Baum M. Lymphoedema, prevention rather than cure. *Ann Oncol* 1991;2:532–33.
7. Casley-Smith JR. Modern treatment of lymphedema. *Mod Med* 1992;35(5):70–83.
8. Brennan MJ. Lymphedema following the surgical treatment of breast cancer: a review of pathophysiology. *J Pain Symp Manage* 1992;7(2):74–80.
9. Rogers TF, Bauman LJ, Metzger L. An assessment of the Reach to Recovery program. *CA Cancer J Clin* 1965;35:116–24.
10. Rinehart ME. The Reach to Recovery program. *Cancer* 1994; 74(1):372–5.
11. Knobf TK. Symptoms and rehabilitation needs of patients with early stage breast cancer during primary therapy. *Cancer* 1990;66:1392–401.
12. Miller LT. Postsurgery breast cancer outpatient program. *Clin Manage* 1992;12(4):50–7.
13. Stumm D. Considering the whole woman: rehabilitation of the breast cancer patient. *Clin Manage* 1992;12(4):62–7.
14. Wingate L, Croghan I, Nataraja N, Michalek AM, Jordan C. Rehabilitation of the mastectomy patient: a randomized, blind, prospective study. *Arch Phys Med Rehab* 1989;70: 21–5.
15. Brennan MJ, Weitz J. Lymphedema 30 years after radical mastectomy. *Am J Phys Med Rehab* 1992;71(1):12–4.
16. Aitken DR, Minton JP. Complications associated with mastectomy. *Surg Clin N Am* 1983;63(6):1331–52.
17. Clarysse A. Lymphoedema following breast cancer treatment. *Acta Clin Gelgica* 1993;15:47–50.
18. Swedborg I. Volumetric estimation of the degree of lymphoedema and its therapy by pneumatic compression. *Scand J Rehab Med* 1977;9:131–5.
19. Boris M, Weindorf S, Lasinski B. Lymphedema reduction by noninvasive complex lymphedema therapy. *Oncology* 1994; 8(9):95–110.

20. Mirolo BR, Bunce IH, Chapman M, Olsen T, Eliadis P, Hennessy JM, et al. Psychosocial benefits of postmastectomy lymphedema therapy. *Cancer Nurs* 1995;18(3):197–205.

21. Zeissler RH, Rose BG, Nelson PA. Postmastectomy lymphedema: late results of treatment of 385 patients. *Arch Phys Med Rehab* 1972;53:159–66.

22. Richmond DM, O'Donnell TF, Zelikovski A. Sequential pneumatic compression for lymphedema: a controlled trial. *Arch Surg* 1985;120:1116–9.

23. Yamazaki A, Idezuki Y, Nemoto T, Togawa T. Clinical experiences using pneumatic massage therapy for edematous limbs over the last 10 years. *Angiology* 1988;38:154–63.

24. Földi E, Földi M, Weissleder H. Conservative treatment for lymphedema of the limbs. *Angiology* 1985;35:171–8.

25. Morgan RG, Casley-Smith JR, Mason MR, Casley-Smith JR. Complex physical therapy for the lymphedematous arm. *J Hand Surg* 1992;11(4):437–41.

26. Boris M, Weindorf S, Lasinski B. Persistence of lymphedema reduction after noninvasive complex lymphedema therapy. *Oncology* 1997;11(1):99–114.

The Treatment of Lymphedema

Ethel Földi, M.D.

Foldiklinik, Fachklinik für Lymphologie, Hinterzarten, Germany.

BACKGROUND. Before the treatment of arm lymphedema after breast carcinoma treatment with complex decongestive physiotherapy can be initiated, it is mandatory to differentiate between benign and malignant forms (due to relapse) and to establish the diagnosis of accompanying diseases, if present.

METHODS. In benign lymphedemas, the aim of complex decongestive physiotherapy is to restore the symptom free "Stage 0 of latency" and to maintain fitness for work. The palliative treatment of malignant lymphedemas results in the amelioration of the quality of life.

RESULTS. The results of treatment depend on the experience of the physician in clinical lymphology, on the training and dedication of the lymphedema therapist, and on the compliance of the patient.

CONCLUSIONS. A study concerning gene expression has shown that complex decongestive physiotherapy influences the pathological alterations of the interstitium in lymphedema patients. *Cancer* **1998;83:2833–4.**
© *1998 American Cancer Society.*

KEYWORDS: lymphedema, complex decongestive physiotherapy, manual lymph drainage, inflammation.

Presented at the American Cancer Society Lymphedema Workshop, New York, New York, February 20–22, 1998.

Address for reprints: Ethel Földi, Prof., M.D., Földiklinik GmbH & Company KG, Fachklinik für Lymphologie, Rosslehofweg 2-6, 79856, Hinterzarten, Germany.

Received July 2, 1998; accepted August 20, 1998.

Lymphedema is not a symptom, as other edemas are, but a disease, arising as a consequence of a low output failure of the lymphatic system. A rational therapy must be based on the knowledge of pathophysiology. Progress achieved in the fields of microcirculation and molecular biology enables us to understand many aspects of those morphologic and functional alterations that take place in the tissues as a consequence of lymphostasis.

Due to the increase in the number of patients suffering from lymphedema, the importance of clinical lymphology increases world wide. There are several reasons for this: 1) There are more elderly people. With age, the force of the lymph pumps decreases, and lymphedema risk factors, such as heart failure, diseases of metabolism, and arthropathies, arise. 2) The progress in the treatment of malignancies results in longer remissions and even in more patients cured; however, as a side effect of the therapies, the cases of lymphedema of the head, limbs, and genitalia increase. The method of choice for the treatment of lymphedema is complex decongestive physiotherapy (CDP).

CDP must be embedded into comprehensive medical care: the majority of lymphedema patients suffer from one or even several accompanying diseases. In addition, the results of CDP depend to a very high degree on the stage at which the treatment begins. To prevent harmful side effects, the constituents of CDP often have been applied in a modified form.

Whether lymphedema is primary or secondary has no relevance concerning CDP. Along with the question of accompanying diseases, the main problem is to distinguish between benign and malignant lymphedema: The malignant forms are caused either by untreated carcinoma or by a relapse after carcinoma treatment.

CDP is a tetrade: Its constituents are manual lymph drainage (MLD), skin care, compression, and remedial exercises. MLD applied in an isolated form is absolutely inadequate. In the drainage area bordering the lymphostatic region, mild strokes are applied. The aim is to stimulate lymphangiomotoric activity. Inside the lymphedematous region itself, the strokes are applied with more pressure to limber up indurated tissues. Compression bandages are constructed in the following manner: For skin protection, one pulls on a cotton sleeve. One inserts upholstering materials with either a smooth surface or a rugged surface followed by textile elastic compression bandages.

By using remedial exercises, one activates the muscle and the joint pumps. The aim of skin care is to prevent mycotic and bacterial infections. Skin care starts with hygienic measures. If necessary, disinfective agents are applied; eventually, antimycotics and/or antiallergics are used. In addition to CDP, other methods of physiotherapy often are applied to mobilize joints, to improve the function of the muscle and joint pumps, to rebuild muscles, or to alleviate pains.

CDP is a two-phase treatment. The aim of phase one is to mobilize edema fluid and to initiate the regression of fibrosclerotic tissue alterations. During phase one, the patients need both mentally and physical rest. Treatment must be applied at least once a day and, eventually, twice a day. Uncomplicated cases can be treated as outpatients, and more severe cases are treated as inpatients. Phase two serves to prevent the reaccumulation of edema fluid and to continue the breakdown of the scar tissue.

Phase two is an outpatient treatment. Its main constituent is compression by elastic stockings or sleeves. Self-treatment includes skin care and remedial exercises; if necessary, MLD is applied. The intensity of application of the components of CDP in its two phases depends on the stage of lymphedema at which the treatment starts and on the nature and severity of accompanying the disease.

The palliative treatment of malignant lymphedemas consists of the application of phase one of CDP. In contrast to the treatment of benign lymphedema in which diuretics have no place whatsoever, in malignant lymphedema, CDP often must be complemented with diuretics. In contrast to benign lymphedema in which CDP serves to maintain the patient's fitness to work, the role of CDP in the treatment of malignant lymphedema consists in improving the quality of life.

The prerequisites of successful CDP are the following: 1) What concerns the physician, i.e., knowledge of lymphology and of the pathophysiology of those diseases that are linked to disturbances of microcirculation. A thorough check-up and therapy of accompanying diseases are mandatory. 2) Physiotherapists must be trained both by clinical lymphologists and by experienced physiotherapists. They must have a deep insight into anatomy and into the consequences of surgical and irradiation therapy of carcinoma. They must be aware of the contraindications of CDP and its various modifications. 3) The materials for bandaging and compression stockings, i.e., sleeves made to measure, must be available in excellent quality. 4) Full compliance of the patient is mandatory. If the patient is not ready to wear the compression stockings, then relapse will occur. Also, if CDP fails, the possibility of self-mutilation, which is by no means rare, must be taken into consideration.

Unfortunately, there is a world wide ignorance concerning the clinical symptomatology of lymphedema. Consequently, false forms of treatments are initiated. This statement can be illustrated by an example. A couple of days ago a 32-year-old man was sent to me. His disease has been initiated by a minor accident involving the right hand while making pizza. Soon, an elephantiastic, very painful lymphedema of the right arm arose. Later on, both lower extremities became lymphedematous as well. The diagnoses of several doctors and hospitals included lymphedema of the right arm, chronic pain syndrome, and generalized reflectory sympathetic dystrophy syndrome.

The treatment consisted in the intrahecal application of morphine with a pump. Amputation of the arm had been recommended. It was a case of self-mutilation: The young man constricted his limbs with bands. His motive was to obtain an invalid pension.

I would like to stress that benign lymphedema does not cause pain, and generalized reflectory sympathetic dystrophy syndrome does not exist. In this case, CDP will not work; the patient must be entrusted to a psychiatrist.

It is generally known that the tissue alterations in lymphedema correspond to a chronic inflammation. In a clinical study not yet published, we have shown that phase one of CDP of a duration of 4 weeks significantly reduces the gene expression of CD14, VLA4, TNFR1, and CD44. This means that CDP reduces or alleviates the chronic inflammatory process. Our findings provide an explanation for the regression of the fibrosclerotic tissue in the course of phase two of CDP.

American Cancer Society Lymphedema Workshop

Supplement to **Cancer**

The Physical Treatment of Upper Limb Edema

Oliver Leduc, P.T.[1]
Albert Leduc, Ph.D.[1]
Pierre Bourgeois, M.D.[2]
Jean-Paul Belgrado, P.T.[1]

[1] Academic Department, Physical Therapy, University of Brussels, Brussels, Belgium.

[2] Nuclear Medicine Service, St. Pierre Hospital, Brussels, Belgium.

BACKGROUND. Edema of the upper limb, without any doubt, constitutes the most invalidating complication of breast carcinoma treatment. The swelling of the limb results from decreased liquid evacuation by surgical intervention at the axillary level and also by the eventual treatment by cobaltotherapy.

METHOD. The physical treatment for edema of the limb consists of a combination of therapies that were tested for their effectiveness in laboratories on healthy students and also on patients who underwent surgery for breast carcinoma. The treatment consists of the application of manual lymphatic drainage (type Leduc), the use of multilayered bandages, and the use of intermittent pneumatic compression. The population studied was represented by 220 patients who underwent breast surgery. The authors followed their evolution during the first 2 weeks of treatment. Patients were not hospitalized. The edema was measured by using marks tattooed on the skin.

RESULTS. The limb that developed edema was compared with the healthy limb. The most important reduction was obtained in the first week. The decrease was equivalent to 50% of the average of the difference between both upper limbs. During the second week, the results obtained stabilized; however, there was a slight decrease at the end of the second week.

CONCLUSIONS. The physical treatment of edema represents the preferred therapeutic approach. However, it must answer to well-defined criteria to be efficient and for long-lasting effects. The physical treatment is used to treat outpatients, allowing them to follow a normal lifestyle. *Cancer* **1998;83:2835–9.**
© *1998 American Cancer Society.*

KEYWORDS: physical treatment, edema, breast carcinoma, manual lymphatic drainage, pneumatic compression, upper extremities.

Lymphedema is characterized by the concentration of proteins caused by various physiopathological processes and, especially, by the lowering of protein resorption. So long as the proteins stagnate in the interstitial spaces, the osmotic pressure remains at a high level, and the edema is maintained. This is quite disturbing, because the protein concentration will favor the fibrous organization of the edema and will act as a stimulus, causing chronic inflammatory processes. Physical therapeutic treatment is the appropriate technique for treating edema of the upper limb. Experience has proven that the physical techniques we use are not limited to symptomatic treatment of the disease but, in many ways, are the most curative treatments.[1]

Even if we insist on the necessity of an accurate diagnosis, treatment, on the other hand, is initiated based on clinical signs. These signs plus the anamnesis of the edema provide sufficient information to allow the expert practitioner to change or vary the physical treatment.

We will restrict ourselves to discuss only the physical techniques that are most appropriate in relation to insufficient drain-

Presented at the American Cancer Society Lymphedema Workshop, New York, New York, February 20–22, 1998.

Address for reprints: Oliver Leduc, P.T., Service de Kinésithérapie et Réadaptation, C.P. 168, 50 Avenue F.D. Roosevelt, 1050 Brussels, Belgium.

Received July 2, 1998; accepted August 20, 1998.

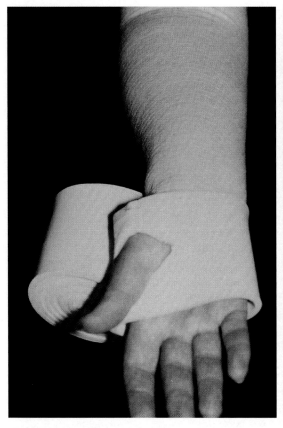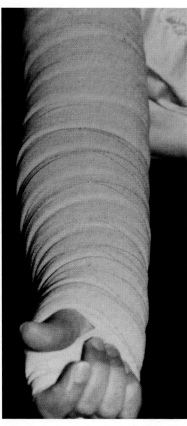

FIGURE 1. Photographs of the cotton tube stretch and latex bandage (left) and the low-stretch bandage (right).

age of the upper limb. The conservative (or physical) treatment is not at all contradictory to the surgical treatment: it is the first step in treatment, whereas surgery is the final step.[2] Conservative treatment can be prescribed from the first signs of edema.

MATERIALS AND METHODS
Manual Drainage
Every treatment by manual lymphatic drainage (MLD) is adjusted to the individual patient. The rules we outline are a guide to proper treatment. Essentially, the therapy depends on the particular reaction of the edema in each patient. The absolute rule not to be broken is this: The manipulation must always be very superficial and extremely soft.[3] MLD is effective only if there are still some lymphatics left, so that they can be activated,[4] and an appearance or an increase of infiltration can be stopped.

MLD itself rarely is sufficient to evacuate edema. Thirty years of experience have shown that improvement can be maintained over the years if certain precautions are taken (i.e., prophylaxy of edema). MLD is applied without any other technique when the volume of edema is very restricted during the first period of edema formation.

Generally, MLD will be only a part of the total

edema treatment. Our experiments demonstrate that MLD stimulates the resorption of proteins.[4] This way MLD is part of the global therapeutic approach, as described below.

Intermittent Pneumatic Pressure
Our experiments have shown that pressotherapy essentially influences the resorption of fluids, but rarely, if at all, does it affect the resorption of proteins.[5-7] Pressotherapy alone should never be used, but it is always used in conjunction with MLD. The pressure exerted never exceeds 40 mm Hg: Lymphatics collapse with pressure that is any greater.[3] Manual and mechanical pressure depends on the physiological conditions of the evacuation by stimulation of the still existing lymphatics. Intermittent pneumatic pressure (IPT) is applied for 1 hour.

Multilayered Bandages
The bandages used in the treatment of lymphedema (see Fig. 1) behave as a nonelastic envelope. Muscle contractions cause pressure in the limb, and the inner pressure varies as a result of changes in volume related to the contraction intensity.[8] If we apply a rigid bandage around the limb, then the effect of the contractions will increase considerably in the limb.[8]

There is probably some relation between the effect of the pressure and the mechanical quality of the dressing. Thus, a nonelastic tissue that is resistant to stretching during muscle contraction undoubtedly will receive higher pressure than an elastic tissue that allows stretching.

The massage effect can be defined as the difference between maximum and minimum pressure values at the borderline of skin and bandages during muscle activity.[8,9] We studied several bandages in laboratory situations on simulated limbs as well as on patients. Superposition of several bandages, as in the case of multilayered bandages (MLB), results, at the borderline of skin and bandages, in pressures lower than when the normal elastic bandages are used.[9] The use of MLB increases the lymph flow.[10] Isodynamic muscle contraction under MLB results in a significant increase in the resorption of the edema. These experiments all involved the upper limbs.

A cotton tube stretch bandage embraces the limb, protecting the skin against full contact with the latex bandage (Fig. 1, left; type Komprex Binde; Lohmann). The latex bandage is placed so that it is half-covering the limb without any tension. The nonelastic bandages (Durelast; Lohmann) also are applied on the limb from the distal region toward the proximal region (Fig. 1, right). Note that we used several bandages, so that we could apply them in a criss-cross pattern to provide axial rotation of the whole MLB. The application of the MLB ended proximally.

Measurements

We used tattooed reference markings on the patient's skin. These markings were localized at 20, 30, 40, 50, and 60 cm from the distal extremity of the middle finger. Perimeter measurements were taken before each treatment during the first 2 weeks.

The patients were treated five times per week. Each treatment lasted 2 hours. Measurements were taken on the side of the edema and on the healthy side. The different values for each limb were totaled and then divided by the number of measures (5 measures). The averages of the difference between the 2 values were compared (Fig. 2). This statistical study was limited to the first 2 weeks of treatment (10 treatments): The treatment during these 2 weeks was followed by another treatment in which the permanent, custom-made sleeve replaced the MLBs.

Population

The population consisted of 220 women who underwent surgery for breast carcinoma (one breast). The patients' ages ranged from 35 to 77 years. The patients were not hospitalized and they led normal, everyday

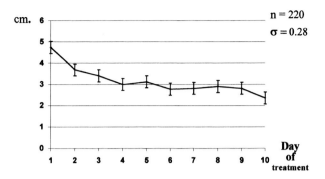

FIGURE 2. Average of the difference between healthy arm and edematous arm.

lives. Follow-up was organized over several months and even several years. However, the statistical study was limited to the first 2 weeks of physical treatment. No medicine had been administered to the study population.

RESULTS

The most important reduction in the edematous limb was registered during the first treatment week and, more specifically, on the second day (Fig. 2). This important decrease between the first and second treatment undoubtedly is the result of massive elimination of fluids by the veins. This hypothesis is confirmed by the fact that patients who present with heart failure withstand a little more difficulty on this first day treatment. The reduction observed at the end of the second week (10th treatment), compared with the fifth treatment, is significant but is relative to the results obtained (Fig. 3a–c). It is at this time that we modified the treatment by replacing the MLB with a custom-made, low-stretch elastic sleeve.

CONCLUSIONS

The measurements obtained from the first treatment show a very important reaction of the edema in association with these different therapeutic approaches used simultaneously. This first therapeutic step is followed by another during which the MLB is replaced by a custom-made sleeve. This sleeve, at first, is worn day and night and then only during the day. On the other hand, the MLD and IPT treatment is administrated five times weekly and diminishes progressively to twice weekly, then once weekly, and finally is discontinued. Certain patients are treated once more after several months, once a week, to maintain results (Fig. 3d). In the majority of cases, the treatment can be interrupted after a progressive decrease of the treatment frequency. However, we must take into consideration that, in accordance with the handicap gravity

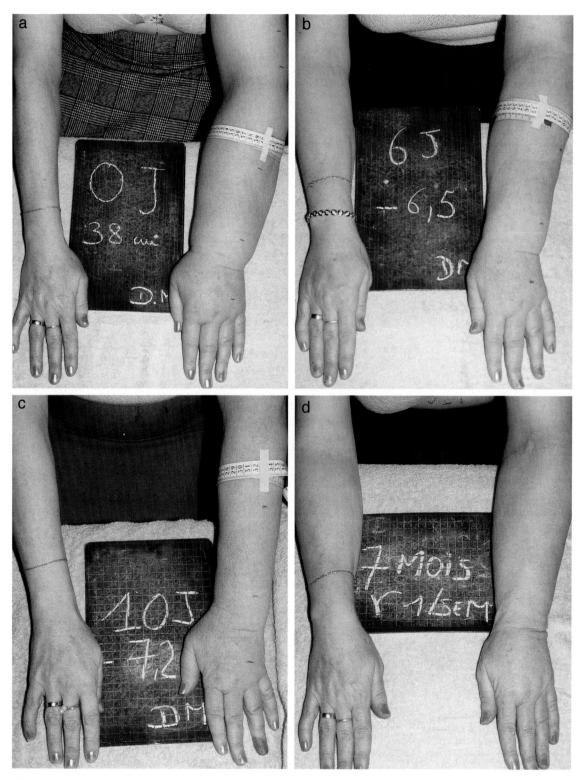

FIGURE 3. Photographs showing edema of the upper limb postmastectomy in one patient before treatment (a), after 6 days (b), after 10 days (c), and after 7 months (d).

of drainage (veinous and lymphatic), certain patients will have to undergo treatment for several months to maintain the results acquired during the first 2 weeks.

Finally, results show that the edema has never totally disappeared. It is exceptional to reduce the edema entirely and to return the treated limb to its healthy

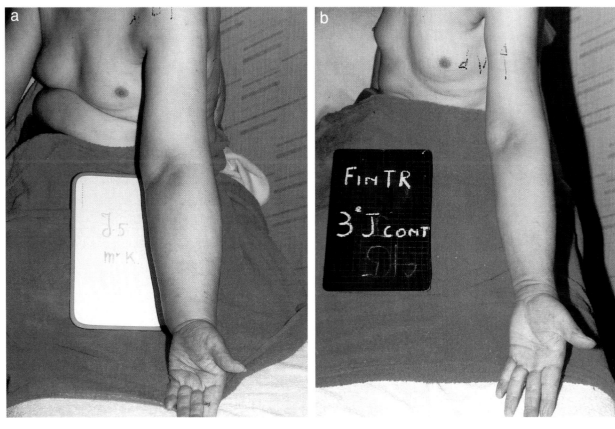

FIGURE 4. Photographs showing the upper limb after axillar adenectomy in a male patient with breast carcinoma before (a) and at the end of (b) treatment.

state aspect (Fig. 4a,b). Generally, upper limb edema is reduced significantly, but a difference in the two limbs remains noticeable when both limbs are placed side by side. One of the essential aspects of the therapy is that the patients studied have not received any medication, and none of them has been hospitalized for physical treatment. This physical therapeutic approach allows the patients to be treated while benefiting from a normal professional, social, and family lifestyle.

REFERENCES

1. Leduc A, Caplan I, Lievens P, Leduc O. Le traitement physique de l'oedème du bras. In: Monographies de Bois-Larris. Paris: Masson, 1991.
2. International Society of Lymphology Executive Committee. The diagnosis and treatment of peripheral lymphedema [consensus document]. *Lymphology* 1995;28:113–7.
3. Eliska O, Eliskova M. Are peripheral lymphatics damaged by high pressure manual massage? *Lymphology* 1995;2: 21–30.
4. Leduc O, Bourgeois P, Leduc A. Manual of lymphatic drainage: scintigraphic demonstration of its efficacy on colloïdal protein reabsorption. In: Progress in lymphology IX. Excerpta medica. Partsh, editor. Amsterdam: Elsevier, 1988.
5. Leduc A, Bourgeois P, Bastin R. Lymphatic resorption of proteins and pressotherapies. Vième Congrès group. Européen de Lymphologie (G.E.L.). *Porto* 1985;31:5.
6. Leduc O, Dereppe H, Hoylaerts M, Renard M, Bernard R. Hemodynamic effects of pressotherapy. In: Progress in lymphology XII. Excerpta medica. Nishi, et al., editors. Amsterdam: Elsevier, 1990:431–4.
7. Partsch H, Mastbeck G, Leitner G. Experimental investigations on the effect of a pressure wave massage apparatus (Lympha Press®) In: Lymphedema, Phlebologie und proktologie. 1980.
8. Leduc O, Klein P, Demaret P, Belgrado JP. Dynamic pressure under bandages with different stiffness. *Vasc Med* 1993; 466–8.
9. Demeyer D, Klein P, Vandeput D, Leduc A, Demaret P. Etude comparative du comportement de bandages élastiques et non-élastiques utilisés dans le traitement de l'oedème lymphatique. *Ann Kinésithérapie (Paris)* 1988;15: 461–7.
10. Leduc O, Peeters A, Bourgeois P. Bandages. Scintigraphic demonstration of its efficacy on colloïdal protein reabsorption during muscle activity. In: Progress in lymphology XII. Excerpta medica. Nishi, et al., editors. Amsterdam: Elsevier, 1990:421–3.
11. Mislin H. Experimenteller Nachtweiss der Autochtonen Automatic der Lymphgefasse. *Experientia* 1961;17:29–32.
12. Leduc A. Le drainage lymphatique. Paris: Masson, 1980.

The Vodder School: The Vodder Method

Renato G. Kasseroller, M.D.

The Vodder School, Walchsee, Austria.

BACKGROUND. The history and development of manual lymphatic drainage (MLD) from Winiwarter to Vodder and the Vodder School of today are discussed.

METHODS. The Vodder technique differs in the use of adapted pressure and its application. The constant change in pressure optimizes results, moving fluid in the skin, increasing lymphomotoricity, and softening fibrosis, with the positive side effects of reducing pain and relaxing tense muscles. Another difference from other methods is the technique of stretching skin, not sliding it. Because of the fluid content in lymphedema, which is different from all other edemas, the combination of MLD with compression treatment is the only solution for this pathology. Depending of it severity, each case requires individualized treatment. Phase I (intensive treatment) consists of daily treatment with up to two sessions per day for up to 2 hours. This phase is combined with special, individual skin care and remedial exercise. In phase 2, the goal of treatment is to maintain the results achieved in phase 1. The frequency of treatment is changed, but there is still the need for permanent, continued therapy.

RESULTS. In phase 1, an average reduction of more than 40% of edema volume is achieved. In phase 2, the results are maintained and, with repetitions of phase 1, further improvement is possible. Thus, long term results with permanent improvement are possible.

CONCLUSIONS. Because of the complexity of the technique, no one can learn MLD in 1 week. Students require a great deal of correction, and the technique must be checked constantly. To become a certified Vodder therapy, a 4-week education program must be completed, and reviews must be attended every 2 years to maintain certification. The best education produces the best results for patients as long as patients are compliant. Therefore, the Vodder School also includes a patient education program as part of its curriculum. *Cancer* **1998;83:2840–2.**
© *1998 American Cancer Society.*

KEYWORDS: manual lymphatic drainage, compression treatment, lymphomotoricity, the Vodder School.

The Vodder School, which started in Germany in the 1960s and then expanded to Austria, was the original school for manual lymphatic drainage (MLD) and, later, for combined decongestive physical therapy as well. Together with Dr. Vodder; the founders of the school, Günther and Hildegard Wittlinger, and physicians from different German Universities developed the modern technique of MLD. Vodder employed circular strokes in different varieties. In the 1960s and early 1970s, the founders of the school adapted these strokes to be modern edema technique,[1,2] and, along with the edema technique, they combined treatment with compression because of the pathophysiological nature of edematous tissue based on scientific works by Professor Hutzschenreuter. The school bears Vodder's name but uses and teaches modern techniques. The strokes that Vodder adapted after

Presented at the American Cancer Society Lymphedema Workshop, New York, New York, February 20–22, 1998.

Address for reprints: Renato G. Kasseroller, M.D., The Vodder School, Alleestraase 30, A-6344 Walchsee, Austria.

Received July 2, 1998; accepted August 20, 1998.

new research are only part of the lymphedema management program.[3]

In 1892, in Billroth's book of German surgery, Winiwarter from Brussels described the four legs of lymphedema treatment: massage with very light pressure (from proximal to distal), nonelastic bandaging, special skin care, and exercises.[4] Now, we call it complex physical therapy or complex decongestive therapy, bit it is very old, and MLD (the decongestion) is a part of it. With every kind of massage, there will also be some decongestion caused by increased tissue pressure. There will be better resorption, but that is not everything; resorption caused by tissue pressure is the lesser part of efficacy. We also move the fluid in the connective tissue; but the most important result of the drainage is the activation of the lymphangion, the increased motoricity of lymph vessels, which was demonstrated by Mislin in the 1970s.[5]

We work with a very light pressure that is adapted to the different tissues and pathology. After a fresh injury, the pressure used is extremely light. In fibrotic tissue, we work with greater pressure, but not too much, to avoid redness. We do not slide over the skin: we push and stretch the skin in two different phases of our strokes. After this, we have a relaxing phase in which no pressure is applied, but there is perfect contact with the skin ("the weight of a fly is to much"). This is one of the most important problems for students and needs a great deal of care and attention from the instructors. The permanent change in pressure, from pushing to zero pressure, creates the pumping efficacy. This change in pressure is in all the strokes. The skin is stretched; we do not slide along.[6] The direction of the push and pressure depends on the direction of lymphatic flow in the skin. We always work with the hand, the only exceptions being the fingers; the handwork creates the push.

It is important to allow enough time, because the strokes must be repeated. The rhythm and the monotone strokes influence the vegetative system, creating a sympathicolytic effect. Today, we know a great deal about connective tissue, flow, retention of fluid, proteins, and histologic structure. In particular, the research from Castenholz gave new information about the architecture of lymph vessels. There is suction at work by the lymph vessels. Some parts of the flow can be reached with external pressure, but we do not move all of the fluid, especially not the proteins. Also, if the proteins are left, the fibrosclerotic changes, then the induration is started.

We educate physical therapists, massage therapists, occupational therapists, and registered nurses in lymphedema management—only those with basic medical knowledge—and the techniques are based on

TABLE 1

The Vodder School Curriculum: Manual Lymphatic Drainage Course and Lymphedema Management (Medical class)

First session
  Introduction
  Physiology of the nervous system, gate control, immunological system
  Histology and physiology of connective tissue, body fluids, contents
  Physical and chemical transportation
  Anatomy of blood vessels and lymph vessels
  Histology of lymph vessels
  Contraindications
Second session
  General pathology: edema, fibrosis, inflammation and infection, wound healing
  Classification of edema and lymphedema
  Classifications of stages of lymphedema
  Basic knowledge for practical treatment with manual lymphatic drainage
Third session
  Primary and secondary lymphedema of arm and leg, had and facial edema
  Cyclic idiopathic edema, lip edema, varicose veins, phlebedema
  Traumatology, rheumatology
Fourth session
  Special indication from neurology, pediatric, dermatology

published research, medical reality, and no hypothesis. Students learn about all of the pathologies that involve lymphostasis and other pathologies in which MLD can be applied because of its decongestive effect on edema. There always seems to be a need for this, because the student's knowledge is sometimes poor in this regard. However, the most important part of the training is the practical education. This complicated manual technique cannot be learned in a few days if perfect results are to be achieved, and perfect results for the patient should be the goal.

In his studies, Hutzschenreuter demonstrated the efficacy of the neuronal structure to the lymph flow.[7] Humans have receptors in the tissue, in the skin, that react through neuronal reflexes to the lymphangions. OUr manual work with these receptors creates increased contractions, and it must be combined with pressure to continue the efficacy. These receptors, which react only to changing stimulation, are different from other receptors, like the noiceptors. They lymphangions work like little hearts: They also have a refractor period, which is another reason for the different pressures used.

Each patient with lymphedema presents a unique, individual case because of the anatomic varieties of the lymphatics and the different surgical techniques. Also, other influences, like radiation or local inflammation, accelerate the pathophysiological alterations. To address all of these problems, we teach our technique and pass on our wide experience.

Depending on the severity of lymphedema, different dosages of treatment are required. Stage 1 edema requires less treatment than stages 2 or 3. With the

TABLE 2
The Vodder School Curriculum—Practice[a]

Week 1
  Basic technique
  Neck-face, scoop technique
  Leg-arms, rotary technique
  Back, nape, loin
  Breast, stomach
  Whole body repeat
Week 2
  Face with special technique, neck (mouth inside)
  Arm with special technique (epicondylitis)
  Leg and special technique (loin and special technique, Cox)
  Nape and special technique (periarthritis)
  Back and special technique
  Stomach and special technique, bandaging I
Week 3
  Repeat bandaging II and III, lymphedema after mastectomy, secondary
    lymphedema leg
  Cranial secondary lymphedema, pathology in head
  Trigeminus, meniere, eyes, Bell's palsy
  Hip, elbow, shoulder
  Abdomen, repeat postmastectomy lymphedema
Week 4
  Secondary leg edema, bilateral mamma, bilateral leg edema
  Burns, ulcer, primary leg edema
  Primary leg edema, mamma, bandaging IV
  Special pathologies
  Final test

[a] The complete course consists of 160 hours.

TABLE 3
Lymphedema Management

Lymphedema management is a combined therapy with active and passive
    treatment by specially educated therapists in two stages
  Stage 1 Improving and decreasing the limb volume by therapists
  Stage 2 Maintaining the results from stage 1 by therapists and self treatment of
    the patients
Treatment
  Assessment by the physician
  Physical examination, measurement, documentation by therapists and/or
    physicians
  Manual lymph drainage
  Bandaging
  Remedial exercises
  Skin care
  Additional medical treatments (e.g., skin care, ulcer treatment)
  Instruction in self bandaging
  Instruction in exercise treatments
  Instruction in nutrition
  Additional psychological advice
  Supervision in additional secondary pathological problems
  Additional physiotherapeutic treatments
  Adapting physiotherapeutic treatments
  Adapting custom-made compression garments
  Wound care program

treatment in stage 1, we prevent more severe pathology. In our hospital, we treat all stages of edema on an inpatient and outpatient basis. We distinguish between two phases of treatment: the intensive phase and the maintenance phase. The intensive phase includes the complete decongestion program with MLD and bandaging twice daily for 45 minutes or more at each session.

Skin care and exercises are applied two or three times daily. Self-treatment instructions and dietary programs are optional. In the maintenance phase, MLD and compression garments or bandaging are used on an individual basis for one session every 2 weeks up to three session per week. In the long term, it is apparent that the earlier treatment starts and the longer it continues, the better and more cost effective are the results achieved. In later stages 2 and 3 of treatment, there should be no more that 15 months between intensive treatment, and the maintenance phase should be a continuous treatment without long breaks.[8]

Tables 1–3 show the training curriculum for MLD and compression therapy. After certification, therapists must attend a review every 2 years. Their technique is checked and corrected, and their knowledge is increased with the latest standards. Only then will they receive recertification from the Vodder School.

REFERENCES

1. Vodder E. Le drainage lymphatique, une novelle methode therapeutique. Paris: Santè pour tous, 1936.
2. Vodder E. Die technische Grundlage der manuellen Lymphdrainage. *Physikalische Therapie* 1983;1.
3. Kurz I. Textbook of Vodder's manual of lymph drainage, vol II. Heidelberg: Haug-Verlag, 1989.
4. Winiwarter F. Die chirurgischen Krankheiten der Haut und des Zellgewebes. Billroth Chr., Deutsche Chirurgie, Lieferung 23. Stuttgart: Verlag Ferdinand Enke, 1892:152–292.
5. Mislin H. Handbuch der allgemeinen Pathologie, 3, Band 6. Teil: Springer Verlag, 1972.
6. Kasseroller R. Kompendium der Manuellen Lymphdrainage nach Dr. Vodder. Heidelberg: Haug-Verlag, 1996:198–209.
7. Hutzschenreuter P, Brummer H. Die Wirkung der manuellen Lymphdrainage auf die Vasomotion. Aktuelle Beiträge zur manuellen Lymphdrainage 19. Heidelberg: Haug-Verlag, 1992.
8. Kasseroller R. The lymphedema and CPT: Proceeding of XVI. ISC Congress, Madrid: 1997.

Treatment for Lymphedema of the Arm—The Casley-Smith Method

A Noninvasive Method Produces Continued Reduction

Judith R. Casley-Smith, Ph.D., M.D.[1]
Marvin Boris, M.D.[2]
Stanley Weindorf, M.D.[2]
Bonnie Lasinski, M.A., P.T.[3]

[1]Lymphoedema Association of Australia, Malvern, South Australia, Australia.

[2]Department of Pediatrics, Cornell University School of Medicine, New York, New York.

[3]Lymphedema Therapy, Woodbury, New York.

Presented at the American Cancer Society Lymphedema Workshop, New York, New York, February 20–22, 1998.

The author thanks the many therapists who provided patient research data, too numerous to name individually, but, in particular, the University of Adelaide; the Lymphoedema Association of Australia; the Adelaide Lymphoedema Clinic; Hamilton Laboratories, Adelaide (for supplying benzopyrones); and GEMINI, France (for the Palmmer 900 mercury device).

Address for reprints: Judith R. Casley-Smith, Ph.D., Lymphoedema Association of Austraila, 94 Cambridge Terrace, Malvern, South Australia, Australia 5061.

Received July 2, 1998; accepted August 20, 1998.

BACKGROUND. This paper gives an outline of the Casley-Smith method for the treatment of lymphedema of the arm. It includes a brief summary of the development of manual techniques and the terminology applied to them.

METHODS. The four principles of this method are skin care, manual lymphatic drainage, compression in the form of bandaging and/or garments, and exercise. The massage techniques, especially where they differ from other schools, are described in some detail, as are the principles that apply in compression and maintenance of reduction in lymphedema.

RESULTS. The results of this method have been analyzed both in Australia and in the United States and are discussed briefly. Mention is made of the benefits of the benzopyrones, which have been used for many years, when added to the above treatment. Both benzopyrones and exercise will produce a continued reduction after the treatment course. They are particularly useful in a less compliant patient. It is stressed that the effect of patient compliance, particularly after treatment, makes a great difference to the ongoing success of the regime.

CONCLUSIONS. A comparison is drawn between the efficacy of various current treatments and their cost. This shows that this combined and conservative method of treatment should be considered before recourse to pumps or surgery. The latter seldom achieve the results of decongestive lymphatic drainage, and, in the long term, they are more expensive. Certain preventive measures may be indicated following, e.g., mastectomies. Prevention of the onset of lymphedema is of extreme importance. However, a return to as normal a lifestyle as possible by the patient is also essential. The earlier treatment begins after the onset of lymphedema, the better the prognosis for the patient. Lymphedema can and should be treated. *Cancer* 1998;83:2843–60. © 1998 American Cancer Society.

KEYWORDS: lymphedema, compression, exercises, benzopyrones, massage, lymphatics, postmastectomy.

The Nature of Complex Physical Therapy—History and Nomenclature

Winiwater was the first to introduce physical therapy for lymphedema.[1] It then fell out of use, why is uncertain, especially because techniques of *lymphatic massage (drainage)* were improved in the 1930s by Vodder.[2] These were modified and extended in practice by Asdonk and Leduc, and later by Földi.

Perhaps the neglect was because Vodder's techniques were directed toward making essentially normal lymphatics work better (e.g., to reduce the edemas of trauma, etc.). They were not designed originally to reduce lymphedema caused by damaged or nonexistent lymphatics—i.e., they did not transfer the lymph to other, still normally drained regions (see below) to the extent that we do now.

Good compression garments were unavailable at that time, and, without these, the reductions produced could not be maintained. Therefore, repeated treatments were necessary. This may have made surgery seem a better option. However, the promises of surgery (reduction operations, lymphovenous or lympholymphatic, anastomoses, and, more recently, liposuction) except in a few special cases, have proved mostly to be disappointing.

By contrast, the recent, very considerable improvements in our knowledge of the detailed anatomy of the lymphatic system by Kubik[3] have allowed many important improvements to be made to the physical therapy of lymphedema, including understanding what is happening and applying this in practice. These improvements have now been refined, improved, and collected into a regimen called *Komplexe physikalische Entstauungstherapie*,[4] literally translated, *complex decongestive physical therapy.*

The work done by the Földis in their clinic and the fact that they published their results finally gave credence to conservative treatment, proving that it was extremely successful in reducing lymphedema and that results could be maintained given patient compliance.[5–7] It was this and the work on the physiology and pathophysiology of the microcirculation and the benzopyrone group of drugs that was done by John Casley-Smith in Oxford and by him, his coworkers in Australia,[8,9] and Földi, as well as that of Kubik[3] on the anatomy of the lymphatic system, that were the most instrumental factors in determining the techniques I have developed for the treatment of lymphedema.

"Decongestive" ("undamming" is the more meaningful, but nonmedical translation) does not have the same connotation in medical English that "Entstauungs" has in German (it makes one think of congestive cardiac failure or some lung diseases). We omit it and use simply "complex physical therapy" (or CPT) to designate this method. We use "physical therapy" rather than "physiotherapy," because this has wider implications internationally and therapeutically. The Földis now often use *"combined physiotherapy."* In a few parts of Australia and the United States, the word "physical" is restricted by law to physical therapists. In such cases, the alternative "complex lymphatic (or lymphedema) therapy" (CLT) is used. It is identical to CPT.

Again, the term "manual lymphatic drainage" (MLD) is copyrighted in the United States and refers to the original Vodder method.[2] Therefore, we refer to "special massage" for the treatment of lymphedema.

Földi has introduced the term manual lymphatic therapy (MLT) for this part of CPT. We (and others) greatly regret this alphabetical confusion, but there is no alternative.

A consensus was agreed upon in New York in February, 1998, in which the Földis, Leduc, the Vodder School (Kasseroller), and Casley-Smith agreed to the term decongestive lymphatic therapy (DLT) as a suitable name for this treatment. We were in total agreement with the four principles involved (see below); however, with the lymphatic massage part of the treatment, there was disagreement on the name. Földi and Casley-Smith opted for MLT. Leduc and the Vodder School opted for MLD. It must be stressed that, although the principles followed are the same for each school of therapy, the massage techniques vary between schools (although parts are very similar). The only way to choose between one another is to evaluate the results of treatment that have been analyzed statistically and published.

CPT for Lymphedema of the Arm
CPT involves four aspects: 1) skin care and the treatment of any infection; 2) a special form of massage; 3) compression bandaging (a garment is prescribed at the end of the course); and 4) special exercises that complement the massage. It has two phases: 1) a treatment course of up to 4 weeks or more gaining the reduction and 2) maintaining and continuing the reduction by continuing with compression, exercises, and skin care.

The massage is based on the concept of emptying the truncal regions first to give the lymph from the periphery somewhere to go; i.e., an empty reservoir is created. Only then is the limb massaged.[3] The proximal region of the limb is always cleared first, then the massage is extended distally. Starting at the distal end and attempting to push the lymph into the unemptied, proximal regions is contraindicated. Other deeper abdominal work may be performed by a well trained therapist that will aid in the clearance of this region and create a larger reservoir for drainage from the thoracic quadrant.

Once a plateau in the reduction is reached, the later massage concentrates on enlarging collateral lymphatics linking obstructed lymphotomes to normal ones. For a single lymphedematous limb, massage and bandaging takes at least 1 hour, but a better result is obtained if a longer time is spent.

A course is repeated after the body's connective tissue has been given time to remodel into its new, less edematous shape. Even the loose skin remodels. This happens fairly slowly, taking 6–9 months. For this reason, courses usually are spaced 1 year apart. They are repeated as often as necessary. Each repetition usually results in the removal of about 50% or more of the edema remaining after the previous course.

Repetition courses will not be necessary if the arm has been reduced to the normal size by the first course of treatment and if the patient is compliant, wears their garment, and continues with some self-massage and exercises. When necessary, the length of the course may be reduced to a few days. Of course, this saves both the expense and the patient's and therapist's time. If the therapist is expert enough in the first place, and if patient compliance is good, then a second course should not be necessary with lymphedema of the arm.

There are certain diseases that potentially may cause considerable problems when combined with lymphedema and CPT treatment. It is important to be sure that these are not present before starting physical therapy, because this can move a lot of fluid into the blood quite rapidly. Hence, congestive cardiac failure and renal disease must be diagnosed. It is still possible to treat such people, but care is needed that the venous pressure is not raised too much. This is quite possible with pumps,[10] and CPT is likely to do the same. If CPT is to be performed, then, in the first few days (which is when most of the fluid is moved), it is necessary to watch the jugular venous pressure to make sure that it is not increased by more than 1–2 cm of water.

Similarly, diabetes must be well controlled, and too much pressure must not be used in compression bandages and garments. Of course, this also applies if severe arterial disease is present in the limbs, and if there are lymphovenous shunts or Raynaud's disease. Apart from severe arterial disease, CPT is contraindicated over radiation injuries, angiodysplasia syndrome, occult infection, and venous thrombosis. However, if the areas involved by these can be located specifically, CPT can be used elsewhere, especially on the trunk and alternative limb drainage areas.

Other conditions can worsen lymphedema and should be treated. Obviously, skin conditions of the lymphedematous limb are important, especially infections and other inflammation.

Combined Methods of Treatment
Skin care
Much can be done in the early stages of lymphedema and to a "limb at risk" to prevent skin problems. The skin must be kept supple, moist, and in good general condition. Skin problems can cause a local high-protein edema that adds to the load of an already inadequate or over-burdened lymphatic system.[11] Obviously, trauma to the limb (e.g., knocks; abrasions or cuts; burns, including sunburn; and insect bites) must be avoided carefully and, if they occur, treated.[12] The limb also must be kept spotlessly clean and dried gently and very carefully. A mineral-oil cleanser is less drying and better for the skin than normal toilet soap.

The raised temperature and raised interstitial proteins that are present in lymphedema provide the perfect medium for both bacterial and fungal growth.[13–17] It is of particular importance to check for any fungal infection and treat accordingly. Although this type of infection is found most frequently between toes, it can be spread quite easily, and it is not uncommon for it to develop under the fold of a breast and, thus, to worsen the problem.

Problems of bacterial infection, again, should be dealt with immediately when they occur. They will worsen the condition and can be life threatening. They are treated normally with antibiotics. Most respond to penicillin as long as the patient is not allergic to this drug.

Massage techniques for lymphedema
The length of a treatment course and that of each separate treatment session *should* depend on the needs of the individual patient. However, this may not be possible. It may be dictated by a number of factors, e.g., hospital constraints and the availability of therapists. Various constraints of the patient will also affect it, such as money, time available, and travelling distances from the clinic, etc.

The time spent on massage on a consecutive daily basis can range from 40 minutes to 90 minutes or longer per limb involved. If only 40 minutes are available, then at least 30 of these minutes should be spent clearing the trunk and the lymphotomes adjacent to the affected limb in the initial stages. This will produce a much better result than spending more time on the limb itself. If a longer treatment time is possible, then up to 1 hour may be spent clearing the trunk, and, of course, the results will be much quicker and better than in the former situation.

After massage, the patient is bandaged with a gauze sleeve, padding, and bandages of low elasticity ("short stretch") commencing at the distal end of the limb. Time must be allowed for bandaging the limb or limbs after treatment (20 minutes are probably minimal for an experienced therapist).

Massage is done on consecutive days over the necessary period rather than two or three times a week over a longer time. The limb needs to be cleaned, and the bandages must be changed and adjusted daily.

The actual length of the treatment period will vary with the severity of the lymphedema, its cause, and the number of limbs and areas of the trunk affected.

Maximum reduction for a single limb should be obtained in 7–10 days if other complications are absent (e.g., a fibrotic cuff caused by previous pressotherapy). The extension of therapy (e.g., 4 weeks) should further promote the enhancement of collateral drainage and the further breakdown of fibrotic tissues.

Good results are much easier to achieve if treatment is commenced as soon as the limb shows signs of swelling. At this stage the tissues are soft, the skin and fascia have not been stretched greatly, excess fibrotic tissue has not formed, and the elastic tissue is still functional. Obviously, the longer the edema or the lymphedema has been present, the more difficult and longer the treatment becomes, and the more often it will need to be repeated. In the early stages of lymphedema, it is really only the excess fluid and protein that need to be removed; the collecting lymphatics need to be assisted and some new collateral drainage needs to be opened. When much fibrosis is present, many new tissue channels must be made through this before any real drainage is possible. The tissue channels will be increased as the fibrotic tissue softens, and more fluid can be moved.

The second course of treatment may or may not be much shorter than the first course. This depends on the condition of the limb and the patient's socioeconomic and even geographic circumstances. If the limb is continuing to reduce on a steady basis, then a second course is not necessary.

It should be pointed out that, as the edema is removed, oxygenation of the tissues is improved greatly. Hence, the skin changes regress: hair follicles and sebacious glands function once more, hair regrows, and the skin becomes thinner and more supple. If there is skin discoloration, then this should return to normal. Other symptoms of lymphedema, such as pain, immobility, stiffness of the joints, paresthesia ("pins and needles"), etc., should also disappear.

This method is particularly good for the treatment of lymphedema. However, the same principles of drainage are of great help in the treatment of any high-protein edema: acute injury, chronic venous insufficiency, and ulcers.

The body has a number of drainage areas ("lymphotomes") with "lymphatic watersheds," i.e., divisions between different lymphatic drainage areas, between them.[3] If the normal drainage of one lymphotome is blocked, then the lymph can drain only into the adjacent lymphotomes. Correct massage causes the collateral lymphatics (in the superficial and deep lymphatic networks) that cross these watersheds to become larger and to carry more lymph to the normally draining lymphotome. It may also cause proliferation of these vessels.

This applies particularly to the trunk, but also to the limbs. A lymphotome of the trunk drains to axillary or inguinal (groin) nodes. If one of these is blocked, then collateral pathways must be established to take the lymph from this lymphotome to the adjacent lymphotomes and, thence, to the intact axillae/groins.

A major part of the rationale of the massage is to force lymph *gently and slowly* across the lymphatic watersheds, dilating the collateral vessels, thus allowing alternative drainage into the collectors of a normal region. Half of the valves of these collectors face in the correct direction; the rest are incompetent because of the lymphedema (see Fig. 1). Hence, this passage across the watershed is relatively easy.

The other function of the massage is to move tissue fluid into the lymphatics[18–20] (the massage makes the initial lymphatics pump)[21] and then along these through their usual collecting lymphatics (with the massage enhancing their pumping),[22,23] through the lymph nodes that are repeatedly emptied. Thus, it removes excess protein from the tissues and the stimulus for formation of fibrotic tissue.[24,25]

In some cases (e.g., when deep lymphatics are blocked), we rely on the very superficial lymphatics to remove the fluid.[26,27] This network has no valves. There is a considerable dermal backflow from deeper, overloaded lymphatics that can be cleared easily to a different and functioning set of nodes through this network. This can be damaged by reduction operations, including liposuction, in which it is excised and removed. It also can be damaged by too much pressure during massage[28–30] or by pumps if they are used with too much pressure, which is often the case. A fibrous cuff often is built up at the proximal end of the limb, thereby constraining any superficial drainage that was available previously from the limb, where the deeper and collecting lymphatics were unavailable for drainage due to surgery and/or radiotherapy. In some cases, this is the only pathway for drainage from the limb. Careful preservation of the network, therefore, is of paramount importance. Massage techniques to increase pumping of deep vessels, therefore, are not indicated when relying on these vessels.

The nodal areas and trunk need to be cleared briefly again and again as the massage proceeds more distally down the limb. When clearing an arm, the therapist needs to return to the proximal areas that have been cleared previously, and these areas must be then cleared through the particular truncal pathways being used for further drainage. To prevent overloading of vessels that are blocked at a more proximal point, drainage to them may be blocked temporarily

FIGURE 1. A diagram of the collateral lymphatics crossing the watershed. In the normal situation (left), some lymphatics have valves pointing one way, and some have valves pointing in the opposite direction. In lymphedema (right), the lymphatics that direct flow out of the lymphedematous lymphotome simply carry more lymph; those that formerly directed flow into it have their flow reversed. Such reversed flow is possible because the deeper collaterals are dilated, and their valves are rendered incompetent. High external pressure (from compressive bandaging) and massage assist in these increased lymph flows. Norm, normal; L/Edema, lymphedema.

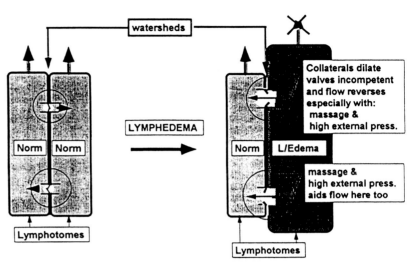

by external pressure with the hand. Then, lymph from the more distal parts is forced gently through the chosen alternative route.

Finally, there may be very hard, fibrotic regions—sometimes forming bands. It is necessary to use a stronger massage pressure to "break" new paths (tissue channels) through these regions. Of course, these channels do not have valves and cannot pump lymph as the lymphatics do. On the other hand, they do allow tissue fluid to pass to regions where true lymphatics exist. (These regions *must* be maintained by graduated compression, because one is usually trying to make the fluid flow upward against gravity.)

The early part of the massage technique concentrates on clearing the adjacent normal regions, increasing pumping by and enlarging the existing collaterals, and softening fibrous tissue, thus reducing the limb. The latter part concentrates on increasing collateral drainage and a greater time is spent on the limb, yielding further reductions. Thus, it is vital to know where blockages have occurred and which are the adjacent, normally draining lymphotomes. Daily circumference measurements help in determining whether one's judgment has been correct.

Massage pressure. This particular type of massage should not cause redness or pain; it is quite gentle. It is stronger when trying to force fluid through sclerotic tissue. The use of excessive pressure can damage the initial lymphatics.[26,30] Learning to use the correct pressures for the lymphatic system is an important part of the training for such a massage.

The initial lymphatics in particular are very fragile. The superficial network lies just below the skin surface. Therefore, a very light pressure will move lymph through these vessels.

Heavier pressure. Heavier but very slowly moving pressure is used when forcing the lymph across a watershed, dilating the collateral lymphatics. A heavier fingertip pressure is also used over the lymph nodes, again with the pressure moving only in the direction of lymph flow.

When deeper pressure is used on fibrotic areas of a lymphedematous limb, this must be counteracted afterward by bandaging firmly. This is to prevent further leakage from the superficial lymphatics whose endothelial junctions may have been opened inadvertently or their endothelium torn during this massage. If, for some reason, bandaging is not being used, then this type of work must be omitted. If it is not, then one will have created leakage of vessels, raised the protein content of the tissues, and probably increased local skin temperatures. These all lead to the possibility of infection and more edema, which will also tend to cause further general swelling. However, such massage cannot be neglected but must be performed with the knowledge of the potential for damage, and care must be taken to counteract it.

These techniques rely entirely on being able to move the hands and fingers over the skin very slowly, with control, and with minimal friction. Therefore, a very fine lubricating talc is used in preference to a lotion, which is too slippery to allow the necessary slowness and control. Normal talcs (even baby powders) usually are not fine enough to allow really precise work. It should be obvious that this massage cannot be performed through clothes or with jewelry either on those areas being massaged or on therapists' hands; otherwise, therapists' senses of touch and of the pressures that they exert can be affected badly.

Clearing the body reservoirs and limbs. The larger lymphatics and nodes of the trunk form a "reservoir" into which the lymphatics of the limb drain. Therefore, the trunk is cleared first to create an empty space into which the lymph from the affected limbs can be emptied easily (it is useless trying to push fluid into a system that is full already). Once this is done, the lymph from the limbs is moved into the reservoirs and on to the previously cleared nodes. If lymph is to be taken from a limb and across the adjacent lymphotome to a normally draining one, then the normal lymphotome is cleared first, then the one adjacent to the limb, and finally the limb itself.

Nodal massage. The lymph nodes are very fine filters distributed along the large collecting lymphatics. Although they are situated throughout the body, they are also clustered at the major points of drainage of both limb and trunk lymphotomes. Because the nodes have 100 times the resistance of the lymph trunks, it is vital to empty these so that they can fill with new lymph. They must be cleared and recleared constantly.

Lymph node massage is performed with the tips of two or three fingers. These are placed over the nodes, and pressure is applied like a gentle "scoop" in the direction of further flow from them. The fingers do not move over the skin; rather, they apply pressure during the scoop and release it, before repeating this several times. It is a slow, deep, but gentle movement. In some areas, e.g., over the deltoid-pectoral ("cephalic") nodes, it could described as a "stationary circle."

The "strokes." This is a light stroking movement over the skin. It is used over the lymphotomes toward previously cleared nodes. This is done with the palm of the hand and the fingers, which are either flat or curved to fit the area being treated. Sometimes, the area is so small that only the distal parts of the fingers can be used.

Relatively small areas are cleared at a time. Therefore, large lymphotomes must be cleared in sections, starting with areas closest to these nodes. When sections that are more distal are reached, these short strokes become longer.

One hand follows after the other to keep the lymph always moving in the desired direction to prevent the possibility of backflow. If therapists position both themselves and their hands correctly, then their fingertips will always end in exactly the correct position to massage the nodes after a few short or longer strokes.

Although mainly short strokes are used, they are followed by longer strokes if the drainage is being taken to nodes at a distance. However, it is the slow work across the watersheds and the continual reclearing of the more proximal areas of the trunk drainage that are most valuable. The whole aim, as emphasized above, are to open new drainage pathways across the watershed through an enlargement of the superficial lymphatic drainage paths and to increase the drainage of the adjacent normal lymphotome through its normal lymphatic system. To do this, half of the deep collaterals crossing the watershed must have their normal direction of flow reversed despite the direction of their valves, and this involves much slow work. The pressure of the "stroke" may be increased slightly as the hand passes over a watershed.

Watersheds. Work over the watersheds is done with a deeper pressure. The ulnar edge of the hand and fifth finger or the widely extended forefinger and thumb move toward and over the watershed in an infinitesimal amount at a time. A constant pressure in the desired direction of lymph flow is maintained throughout.

Flow across watersheds must be enhanced both anteriorly and posteriorly and is performed only after the normally draining lymphotomes have been cleared.

Softening of fibrotic scar tissue. In softening scar tissue the thumbs are often used to break down fibrotic tissues. The pressure is much deeper and is always in the direction of desired lymph flow.

Clearance of deep truncal areas. Deep thoracic clearance can be achieved by a breathing exercise with the patient in a supine position. The patient inhales. On exhalation, the shoulders are "hunched" forward. If it is possible for the patient, the head also may be lifted and the chin pushed forward toward the sternum at the same time.

Deep abdominal clearance during clearance of the ipsilateral lymphotome, when appropriate, also can be achieved by a breathing exercise with externally applied pressure of the therapist's hands to aid with the creation of abdominal pressure (there are situations in which this is contraindicated). Other deeper abdominal work may be performed by a well-trained therapist that will aid in the clearance of this region and create a larger reservoir for drainage from the thoracic quadrant.

Massage sequence. It is essential to perform the massage in an ordered manner to achieve good results, with one hand following the other to keep lymph flowing in the required direction. First, the lymph nodes of the lymphotomes adjacent to the lympho-tome adjoining the lymphedematous limb are cleared. The lymphotomes that drain into these nodes are then emptied. The collateral drainage across the watershed separating these from that adjoining the lymphed-ematous limb is enhanced by very slow work over these areas. Only then is the lymphotome adjacent to the affected limb cleared across the watersheds to the previously cleared lymphotomes and nodes. Having achieved a full trunk clearance both anteriorly and posteriorly, it is possible to start on the most proximal part of the affected limb and to work gradually, after clearance of each section, to the distal regions.

However, it is *vital* that the reservoirs be reemp-tied whenever they become full. A self-aware patient may feel the nodes that drain their limb becoming full; they feel a dull ache. If this happens, then the more proximal reservoirs must be emptied again. In any case, the reservoirs toward which one is working should be emptied many times during a treatment, particularly the nodes.

Massage on nodes or deep vessels that are over-loaded may cause dermal backflow. This can be dealt with by further superficial clearances.

It must be remembered that the four lympho-tomes of the trunk each include all of the thoracic, or abdominal, surface of the trunk from the anterior mid-line to the posterior midline. However, usually, only the anterior and lateral or the posterior and lateral parts of them can be worked at any one time.

Usually, most of the treatment time will be spent on the trunk. For example, if the massage part of a session takes 90 minutes, then the first 60 minutes usually are spent on the trunk alone. As the treatment course proceeds, a longer time may be spent on the affected limb.

It should be pointed out that in a unilateral mas-tectomy, drainage can be taken from the thoracic quadrant and limb of the affected side to both the contralateral thoracic quadrant and the ipsilateral ab-dominal quadrant. However, in the case of a bilateral mastectomy, drainage should always be taken to the ipsilateral abdominal quadrant only. Scar lines or ad-hesions from radiotherapy damage from either of the above operations or from other, totally unrelated op-erations will also determine the pathways that are available for use.

The therapist must realize that these are only guides for treatment pathways and not fixed "recipes." Special attention may need to be paid to particular areas, e.g., a lymphedematous breast or lymphedema in the thoracic area immediately inferior to the axillary area, that manifests as a "bulge." Each patient has

their own individual problems, and the therapist must think and plan the treatment protocols accordingly.

Compression Bandages and Garments

Compression bandages are an essential part of the physical therapy of lymphedema to maintain the re-ductions achieved. Low-elastic (low-stretch) bandages are used to provide compression during the treatment of lymphedema. Compression bandages cause a mild increase in the total tissue pressure,[31–33] and, with exercise, they promote a variation in total tissue pres-sure[34–36] that will increase lymphatic drainage by 1) increasing uptake by initial lymphatics and 2) increas-ing pumping by the lymphangions.

They are particularly necessary in lymphedema, because a feature of this disease is the loss of the elastic fibers from the tissues. They perform a similar function to elevating the limb, reducing the hydro-static pressure gradient from blood to the tissues and increasing that along the lymphatic trunks. They also increase the gradient from the tissues to the initial lymphatics. Their use alone increases lymph flow with exercise and can reduce lymphedema. Graded com-pression, with greater compression distally and lesser proximally, is necessary. A low-stretch bandage plus muscle action will achieve this. It also prevents reflux of fluid back to the precleared, interstitial tissues and prevents further stagnation at the site of the initial lymphatics, so that they are not again overloaded. In the massage part of the treatment phase, this is ex-tremely important. However, to maintain the result obtained by CPT, the graded compression plus exer-cise must continue afterward and be an integral part of the ongoing treatment.

It is very important to distinguish between *elastic* (high-stretch) and *low-elastic* (low-stretch) bandages. Low-stretch bandages are used for compression ban-daging. Elastic bandages have a *high resting pressure* but a *low working pressure.* Not only are they very uncomfortable when the limb is at rest, but they stretch readily when muscles contract—hardly raising total tissue pressure and, thus, lymphatic pumping, at all. *Low-elastic* bandages have a *low resting pressure* and a *high working pressure.* Thus, they supply a com-fortable amount of support to a relaxed limb but in-crease the total tissue pressure considerably when the muscle contract (Fig. 2). The lymphatics are com-pressed between the muscle and the bandage, causing them to pump. The importance of low-stretch com-pression was demonstrated by Partsch and Stem-mer.[37–39]

The lymphatics will pump only when they are compressed (by muscular contraction, massage, or other form of pressure) against something solid and

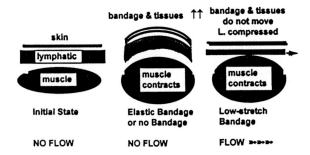

FIGURE 2. This demonstrates the importance of low-stretch bandages for pumping by lymphatics during muscle contraction. On the left is a relaxed muscle with lymphedema between it and the skin. The lymphatics lie in this area. In the center, the muscle has contracted, but the compression garment is either too elastic or nonexistent. The subcutaneous tissue simply moves away from the muscle, there is no compression and no lymphatic pumping. In the right, the muscle compresses the dilated lymphatics between it and a low-elastic compression garment or bandage. This makes the lymphatics pump, and the lymph flows on to the more proximal lymphatics.

unyielding; elastic bandages give way and do not compress the lymphatics, which then do not pump. A bandage with low elasticity (low-stretch) causes a high pressure within the limb when a muscle contracts (the *working pressure*), thus compressing the lymphatics. The *resting pressure*, however, is low [i.e., there is less pressure when the muscles are relaxed than would be the case with an elastic (high-stretch) bandage]; thus, the lymphatics can fill more readily.

During a course of therapy, bandages allow one to reshape a limb much better than garments because of the opportunity to insert various paddings. The bandages should be applied as firmly as is bearable over padding. The padding prevents bandage indentations in the skin and may be thickened to distribute pressure evenly over concave regions.[8]

The radius of curvature is important, e.g., at the sides of the hands, the radius of curvature is much smaller than that of the dorsum of the hand. A single turn of bandage will exert greater pressure where the radius is smaller and far less pressure where it is larger—often just where such increased pressure is most needed. This must be compensated for by extra padding.

The application of multilayer bandaging.
The bandages themselves must be applied with a greater pressure at the distal end of the limb, gradually reducing the pressure toward the proximal end. However, this is achieved by the number of layers and overlap of the bandages. It is *not* done by applying the bandages more tightly at the distal part of the limb. During treatment, a good rule of thumb is that the bandage is applied as tightly as the patient can stand and is comfortable with. If bandages do become tight during the night and pain is not relieved by exercise, the therapist may need to attend and alter them. Fingers are bandaged first, before padding or outer bandaging are commenced.

To obtain an even pressure and as a safety measure to prevent chafing, a fairly low-density foam padding should be used. A "padding" bandage supplements this and evens out the radius of the limb as well as protecting it, before the low-stretch outer bandage is applied. The skin is protected by a washable gauze sleeve, which is changed daily. The padding is used over this (both foam and cotton padding bandages) primarily for protection of the limb against chafing and pressure points. Padding may then be built up as treatment proceeds, and different types of denser foam may be used to make special pads for the softening of fibrotic areas and for reshaping the limb.[8]

A change in bandage width is indicated as the circumference of the limb increases. The number and width of bandages used varies, of course, from patient to patient. The number of bandages needed depends greatly on the pressure of application and also on the particular bandage technique used.

A bandaged limb should feel comfortable. Although flexion at the joints is somewhat restricted, it should be possible for the patient to perform the necessary exercises.

Pressure garments for lymphedema.
Once a reduction of a lymphedematous limb has been achieved, pressure garments[8,49] are essential if the fluid is not to rapidly refill the empty spaces. These cannot be used during the course of the therapy, because the size of the limb is changing so rapidly. Garments must be graded, with the pressure greater distally than proximally.

Availability of the garment is almost as important as efficacy. There is no point in treating a patient by physical therapy and then having to wait weeks for a suitable garment to arrive. Patients often are *not* able to bandage themselves as the clinic does (especially postmastectomy patients). In fact, often, it is hard for them to put on a pressure garment. This means that the choice of bandages and sleeves depends very greatly on good suppliers. If the garment has to be custom made, then, obviously, it is helpful to have a local manufacturer who can do any necessary fine alterations on the spot.

Once a therapist is experienced, they should find that almost all of the reduction occurs in the first 7–10 days, except in complicated cases. When they are confident of this, it means that a suitable fitting garment can be ordered at this point if a made-to-measure garment is required. For this, it is essential that the measurement of the patient in the clinic or by a supplier is done absolutely correctly. Mistakes can be made, but it should not be the patient who has to bear that cost. Measure for a sleeve after a treatment session.

Custom-made garments will not be appropriate for the patient whose condition has not stabilized. Measurements taken on the patient whose edema is fluctuating will not provide accurate information for a well fitting garment. In these instances, or if a patient's therapy has to be delayed, it may be possible to choose a standard compression garment, because these can be fitted at once and monitored for suitability. A custom-made garment, when the measurement for this and the garment supplied are both absolutely correct, invariably is more comfortable. However, standard compression garments are less expensive than a custom-made garment, so this makes them an attractive choice. It is very important, however, to identify those situations in which a standard garment may not be appropriate and may in fact be contraindicated. This is necessary 1) for patients whose circumference measurements show extreme deviations against measurement tables for standard garments (this may result in a tourniquet effect in tight areas and/or a pooling of lymph in loose areas); 2) for patients whose length measurements vary greatly from the average; 3) for awkwardly shaped limbs or deformity; 4) where a nonstandard style is required; and 5) where a nonstandard compression gradient is required.

When choosing a compression garment, the issues of style, material, and compliance also must be taken into consideration. The style of garment will depend on such factors as location of condition (and the need to avoid pooling of fluid either distal or proximal to the garment), age, independence and dexterity of the patient, their life style (active, sedentary, living alone), and work conditions. Environmental factors, such as climate, will influence the wearing of the garment. Suspected poor compliance and/or poor hygiene need to be addressed.

The patient's comfort and, thus, their compliance is of great importance for the maintenance of the progress made during therapy. Much depends on the fit of the garment and the material of which it is made. Some patients have allergy problems to synthetic materials, and a cotton coating of the elastic fibers is then very important; others have the reverse problem. Some garments "breathe" more than others. Some have an inner soft knit. Others can be lined. Anything that gives greater comfort will aid compliance.

A number of patients need gloves or gauntlets. The gauntlet variety (i.e., attached to and part of the sleeve) are preferable, in that they reduce the risk of a pressure band at the overlap. If the lymphedema is severe, particularly in the upper arm, and a good reduction is obtained during treatment, then care must be taken not to prescribe a high-compression sleeve (greater than 45 mm Hg) without an accompanying hand piece. A sleeve to the wrist alone is likely to result in triggering lymphedema of the hand and fingers. However, if the lymphedema is treated in the earlier stages and there is no problem with the hand, then a sleeve from the wrist up is preferable.

One needs to be wary of a sleeve that stops too short of the proximal end of the limb or that causes a pressure band at that (or any other) point. This will *reduce* lymphatic drainage as well as causing a band of fibrotic tissues to form that, later, will also reduce drainage when it contracts.

Many styles and makes are available. When properly prescribed, they are almost equally effective. However, good service and availability from the manufacturer or suppliers may determine which garments the therapist may find most satisfactory for use.

Exercises for Lymphedema

Exercises are an essential part of the CPT program both during treatment and in the maintenance phase. They must be specially designed for patients with lymphedema to be maximally effective. The principle of the exercises that I suggest is to achieve clearance of the trunk and nodes first, so that the affected arm has somewhere to drain to, and then to help clear the arm. They are combined with a certain amount of self-massage, as the program proceeds. The design of these exercises mimics the pattern and massage clearance during CPT.[4]

The exercises are intended as an adjunct to the treatment of lymphedema by CPT. It must be emphasized that they are not intended as a complete treatment of lymphedema by themselves but merely as a most useful addition to existing methods. However, they should also benefit sufferers from lymphedema who, for one reason or another, are unable to attend a clinic. Their effectiveness has been demonstrated not only in improving the results of CPT but in maintaining them.[42,43] To be effective, the exercises must be performed while wearing the appropriate compressive bandaging or compression sleeves or stockings.

Exercises should be taught to the patient when they first start a treatment course. They should be modified to suit each individual patient. Once the patient is competent and able to perform them correctly, it is preferable that they are done at that part of the day furthest removed from their treatment session, because they will act as a separate "minimassage" and an enhancement of lymphatic clearance. The exercises are designed carefully to be followed in sequence. They have five functions: 1) The first exercises empty the more central lymph reservoirs (the nodes and the proximal lymph trunks). Particular attention is paid to emptying adjacent, normal lymphotomes. This provides space into which the lymph from the periphery may flow (otherwise, the very high hydraulic resistance in the nodes reduces the flow of lymph). 2) The remainder of the exercises make any surviving lymphatics work more efficiently. Despite the importance of contractions by the walls of collecting lymphatics, lymph flow is aided considerably by varying total tissue pressure, like what is achieved by the compression of these vessels by contracting muscles against the surrounding fibrous tissues. The initial lymphatics pump *only* by virtue of such varying total tissue pressure. Such variations also greatly assist in the passage of fluid through the interstitial tissue. 3) Exercises help to mobilize joints and swollen areas. 4) Exercises strengthen the muscles of the limb and help avoid muscle wasting, which can be a feature of lymphedema. 5) Exercises are combined with a small amount of self-massage to aid in emptying nodes and the lymphotomes of the trunk.

Adapting the exercises.

Patients, especially elderly, obese, or postmastectomy patients, have varying degrees of movement in their joints. A postmastectomy patient often needs to be encouraged and to have special exercises designed to increase the range of movement in their shoulder joint in order to stop the skin and fascia of the axilla from shrinking. Ideally, these exercises should be taught and supervised after the mastectomy or lumpectomy and radiotherapy (i.e., before there is any suggestion of lymphedema) to prevent deformity and tissue shrinkage. If these have not been done adequately, then mobilization exercises must be taught first before exercises for lymphedema can be performed easily.

Some exercises are difficult, and their correct performance will take some time to achieve. Do not let the patient be disheartened if, at first, the result does not seem quite correct and they cannot feel the muscle or limb section in isolation. This will come with practice.

The exercises need to be modified if a patient has had bilateral mastectomies. Any exercises that push lymph to the opposite side of the chest should be omitted. More time should be spent on those that clear the pelvis on the ipsilateral side. Time should be allowed for nodal and superficial self-massage. This

should be used to clear the superficial inguinal nodes, the lower abdominal quadrants, and, last, the thoracic quadrants across the abdomen to the inguinal nodes. For maximum effect, when possible, these exercises should be performed with the affected limb elevated.

The amount of exercise that should be performed on a daily basis also must take into account the patient's life style and how much exercise they do in the course of their daily work. On days of heavy and unusual work, therapeutic exercises should be lessened accordingly. In fact, a better result may be achieved by doing the trunk clearance exercises only and then lying and resting with the limb elevated for 30 minutes, with periodic flexion and extension of the hand.

Exercise and sport

A patient with lymphedema should avoid exercises or sports that jar the affected limb(s). Tennis may be possible, particularly if a lymphedema of the arm is on the nondominant side. Although caution should be exercised, we do not suggest that a patient give up something that they enjoy doing. If the limb aches after the exercise or sport of their choice, then they should do less of it. Some exercise can help lymphedema, e.g., swimming (but, again, not too much) and scuba diving. Any exercise that a patient finds beneficial is indeed indicated for them; it may not necessarily be of benefit to other patients.

Results of Treatment

The actual results of any form of therapy are most important. These are not only the results immediately after treatment finishes but months to years later. It is clear that the results of CPT are very good indeed—better and faster than any other method of treating lymphedema. However, it must be emphasized again and again that good results depend on a well-trained and careful therapist and on patient compliance after the course. Therefore, a brief summary follows of the results that Casley-Smith-trained therapists have obtained, covering the first course of treatment and ranging from a 1-year to a 3-year follow-up. Informed consent was obtained for the trials described below.

The Adelaide Lymphedema Clinic achieved an average reduction of 64% of the edema over a month's course of treatment for the first consecutive 78 arms to pass through the clinic.[44] The reduction achieved depended on the grade of lymphedema (how much excess fibrosis) and patient compliance. Only a few patients had been treated for more than 1 year, so not so many long term results were available. The results are summarized in Figure 3. Arms were all unilateral. There were very significant differences between the

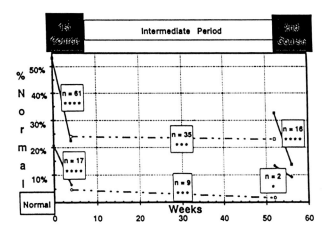

FIGURE 3. Mean values for all arm patients over 13 months. The upper set of lines (squares) refer to Grade 2 lymphedema, and the lower lines (circles) refer to Grade 1. The results of the first and second courses are shown by solid lines, and results of the intermediate periods are shown by dashed lines. Numbers of patients and significance are shown for each period. Because there were fewer patients in each succeeding group, their initial values are different from the final values from the preceding group. It can be seen that well over half of the initial edema was lost in the first course, that this loss not only was maintained but improved slightly during the intermediate period, and that half of the remaining edema was lost during the second course.

grades. Grade 2 lost more liters of edema, but grade 1 lost a greater percentage of edema.

In the first 4-week course of CPT in the arms, the mean grade 1 was reduced from 121% of normal to 107% (a mean reduction of 68%). Grade 2 was reduced from 153% to 123% (a mean reduction of edema of 57%). Over the next year, 44 patients were available to follow. There was a further (nonsignificant) decrease. Another 4-week course in 18 patients resulted in very significant reductions in the residual edema. Even in grade 2 lymphedema in the arms, about 60% of the edema was removed in the first course, and about 60% of the remainder was removed in the second course.

In another trial, the treatment results of over 600 limbs from 22 different therapists[45,46] were analyzed. This was an open trial, but it was the only way this information could be obtained. However, only objective measurements were used, except for patient compliance. Care was taken to obtain results of all patients treated by each therapist. Half of the data were from one clinic alone. No selection was made, and the results of all who received more than 3 days of treatment were included. The effect of CPT and that of a number of factors—exercise, benzopyrones, a mercury pump (Palmmer 900) that was used with a few patients, and patient compliance with garments— were able to be analyzed by multivariate analysis and are summarized in Figure 4–6.

For many years in Australia, many patients have used benzopyrones either alone or as an adjunct to CPT treatment. This paper is not concerned with these trials. However, because, in some trials, both oral and topical forms of these drugs have been an integral part of the treatment, their action must be understood. Benzopyrone drugs reduce lymphedema and elephantiasis. They make the body's macrophages lyse more of the excess protein in the tissues than they normally do. With the protein gone, water can return through the venous capillaries and any functioning lymphatics. The excess fibrosis is removed, and there are far fewer attacks of infection. Hence, they help in all high-protein edemas, including lymphedema.[47-52] Perhaps one of their greater benefits is with patients who may lack compliance after a treatment course, especially regarding exercise. They aid in a continual reduction that would not occur otherwise.

CPT offers great reductions for lymphedema of all grades (including elephantiasis). Older patients improve very significantly more than the younger patients, grade 2 patients improve more than grade 1 patients, and arms improve more than legs. Sex, duration, and cause of lymphedema (including primary lymphedema) make no difference.

However, these reductions are made much greater if benzopyrones are used in association with CPT: oral benzopyrones for at least 3 months before the course of CPT, during, and after it, and topical benzopyrones during and after the course. Reductions also are improved greatly if the patients perform the specifically designed exercises before, during, and after the course. Together, these adjuncts can produce good results even with less skilled therapists; but the more skill, the better the results.

Maintenance of the reduction is also greatly improved by both the oral benzopyrones and the exercises. The compliance of the patient (partly reflected in the care of their compression garments) also is very important in maintaining the reduction.

Although a Mercury compression device, Palmmer 900, assisted reductions for the first course, it did not assist in subsequent courses. Air pumps did not assist at all; indeed, their use was associated with worse results, but this may have been from therapists becoming reliant on these rather than on their own efforts.

The results of the best therapists, of course, are better than those of the average therapist. The therapists from Lymphedema Therapy not only had very intensive and longer training than some of the others but have been able to spend the time necessary with each patient to produce the best results. It is noteworthy that none of their patients needed a follow-up

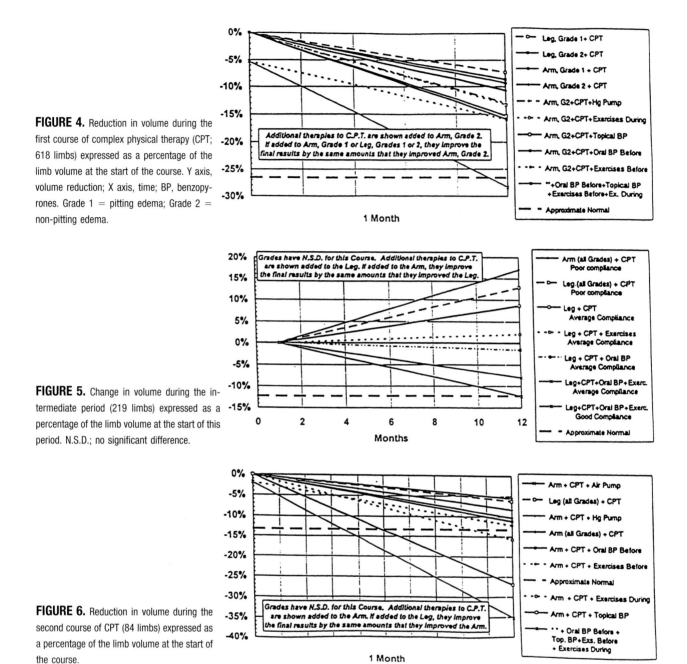

FIGURE 4. Reduction in volume during the first course of complex physical therapy (CPT; 618 limbs) expressed as a percentage of the limb volume at the start of the course. Y axis, volume reduction; X axis, time; BP, benzopyrones. Grade 1 = pitting edema; Grade 2 = non-pitting edema.

FIGURE 5. Change in volume during the intermediate period (219 limbs) expressed as a percentage of the limb volume at the start of this period. N.S.D.; no significant difference.

FIGURE 6. Reduction in volume during the second course of CPT (84 limbs) expressed as a percentage of the limb volume at the start of the course.

treatment and that the degree of good patient compliance was exceptionally high.

Lymphedema Therapy reported 16 arms with a mean reduction of 73%. After 1 year, they had 80% reductions with no further treatment.[52] A later report[53] gives the results of 58 consecutive patients; 56 single arms and 2 bilateral arms. After the first course, reductions were 63% for the unilateral arms. After 3 years, with no further courses, the means for unilateral arms were 64%. Compliance was estimated from the percentage of time the patient wore a compression garment, how they maintained it, and their adherence

to performing the Lymphoedema Association of Australia exercises.[41] For the unilateral arms, patients who were 100% compliant increased their mean reductions from 63% to 79% over the 3 years; the noncompliant patients had their reductions worsened from 63% to 43%. This was highly significant (Figs. 7, 8). All of these results are better than those of the average therapist.

Efficacy of Treatment versus Costs of Treatment

Cost efficacy of CPT compared with other modes of therapy is necessary to consider. For example, many believe that pumps must be cheaper. Both public and

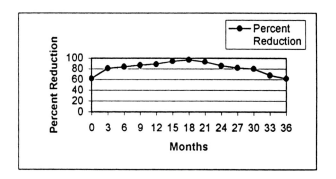

FIGURE 7. Persistence of lymphedema reduction in patients with one lymphedematous arm.

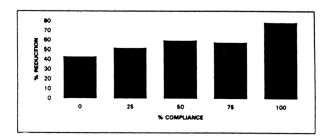

FIGURE 8. Effect of compliance: Reduction in lymphedema in patients with one lymphedematous arm according to the degree of compliance.

private health insurances will often cover the cost of surgery for lymphedema. However, when all factors are taken into consideration, the costs of the above are neither cheaper (and, in the case of surgery, are very much more expensive) than the cost of CPT, and the results are very poor if not negative by comparison.[54]

Whereas the actual costs involved can be calculated, what are impossible to estimate are both public and private costs. These may include having to support a person who becomes disabled, is not able to work or contribute as a taxpayer, or may need disability compensation and perhaps other costly aids to be able to function at all. To this must be added not only the risk, but the cost, of more frequent infections and threat to life in some instances.

The facts that good treatment with CPT can alleviate these problems and that the cost is far less prohibitive than other, unsuccessful, treatments, which may be repeated over many years and, in many cases, may be worse than no treatment at all, must be appreciated and acted upon. The cost of the course of CPT was based on 4 weeks of treatment, and costs of bandages and garments were included (Fig. 9).

These results are expressed only in terms of percentage reductions, because they are measurable. What have not been measured (at least so far) are improvements in the quality of the patients' lives. However, such consideration are far more important

to the patient (and to a responsible doctor or therapist) than mere percentage points.

Although what is affordable (for a patient or a community) ultimately will limit what can be done, some place a higher value than others on returning as closely as possible to normalcy. Thus, again, the individual patient's needs, desires, and geographic and economic circumstances will have to dictate what is done for (and to) them. For many, a treatment far below the "best possible one" is all that can possibly be offered. However, the most important considerations are still whether therapy is available from a well trained therapist for the specific patient, whether they can afford it, and whether they accept the regime and are compliant with it.

Case Histories

The following examples of postmastectomy lymphedema illustrate a number of the different points and provide an immediacy that means and standard errors, however important, cannot convey.

Patient 1

Patient 1 was a 78-year-old woman with postmastectomy lymphedema of the left arm of 17 years' duration. Radiotherapy had caused damage, and the humeral head was showing slow ischemic necrosis. There was also degeneration of the rotator cuff and damage to the distal end of the humerus. She had a greatly restricted range of movement at both shoulder and elbow; for this reason, both the massage and the exercises had to be greatly modified. She could not lie on her stomach; therefore, much of the massage time was spent clearing the anterior parts of the abdominal lymphotomes. There were many scars on the forearm due to the removal of squamous-cell carcinomas (one area measured 1×1.5 cm). These gradually disappeared during treatment with the application of coumarin ointment. The skin was hot, dry, and fragile; it was treated with mineral-oil washes and moisturizers (Hamilton) and with coumarin ointment and powder.

The patient was treated only for 3 weeks because of her age, but the edema was reduced by 55% (Figs. 10–12). She was fitted with a standard Elvarex (Beiersdorf) sleeve. She continued to take oral coumarin and to perform her exercises. There were further reductions in her arm. After 5 months, she could perform normal activities of daily living. After 18 months, she returned for a 2-week course of CPT, achieved a total of 90% reduction in edema (Figs. 13, 14), and is no longer "the lady with the big arm."

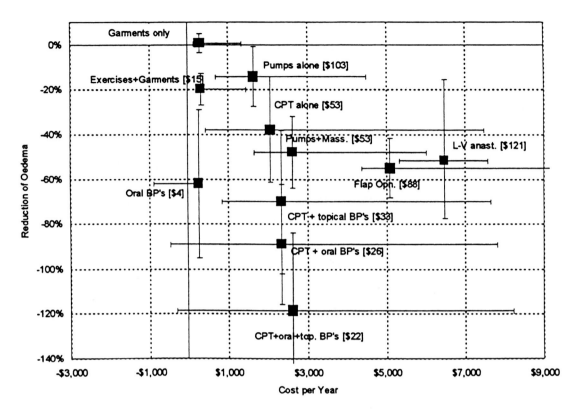

FIGURE 9. Chart of lymphedematous arms showing the percentage reductions in edema over the year and the annual cost of each therapy in U.S. dollars. The reductions are adjusted to allow for the increases of lymphedema that occur if it remains untreated. Average values are shown (square) at the center of a cross formed by the ranges of the best results and the worst results of each for both the percentages and the costs. Labels are as close as practical to each point but, in some instances, had to be somewhat removed onto *one* of the range bars. Following each label is the average cost per 1% reduction in edema per year in brackets. It should be noted that, when benzopyrones (BPs) are used, some of the ranges include negative costs. This is because the costs associated with most of the secondary acute infections are lower, resulting in a total saving of money.

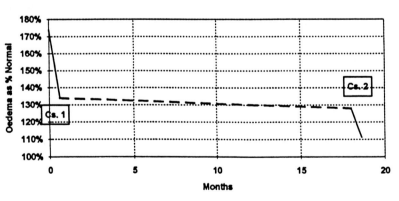

FIGURE 10. Grade 2 postmastectomy lymphedema of 17 years duration (78 years old). The y axis gives the percentage of swelling compared with the normal arm. CPT and oral and topical benzopyrones were used, and exercises were performed. Each course of CPT is shown as a solid line, and the intermediate period is shown as a dashed line. The actual courses are noted by Cs.

Patient 2

An 84-year-old woman had a bilateral mastectomy and axillary dissection and radiotherapy 25 years earlier. Over the next 20 years, there was a gradual increase in edema. She had a history of multiple episodes of cellulitis. She had used a pump for 2 years prior to treatment. The patient's right upper extremity and hand were completely nonfunctional, and she required assistance with all activities of daily living.

On presentation (Figs. 15, 16), she had moderate S.A.I. (secondary acute infection) and was given antibiotics. After this subsided, she was treated with CPT. Initially, the mean circumferential difference was 18 cm greater than the normal arm. After a 3-week course, this was reduced to 4.2 cm, a 77% reduction (Figs. 17, 18). She wore a 20 mm Hg compression garment and had an 83% reduction after 1 month, an 86% reduction at 3 months, and an 89% reduction at 5

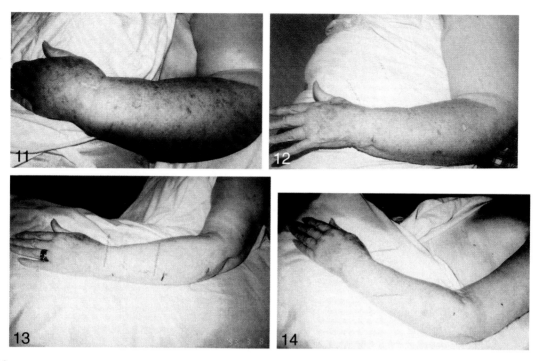

FIGURE 11. Before the first course, note the condition of the skin. Movement was very limited (courtesy of Sydney Lymphoedema practice, P. Dyson and S. Boyce)
FIGURE 12. After the first course, note the reduction and improvement of the skin.
FIGURE 13. Before the second course, the skin and movement were much improved.
FIGURE 14. After the second course, the arm was almost normal, and the skin was excellent.

months (Figs. 19, 20). Her most recent measurement showed a 92% reduction. This again shows how well lymphedema resolves in the elderly.

Relation of CPT to Other Manual Therapies

There are many similarities but also some major differences between the Casley-Smith method and the physical methods of other schools. In each case, the various physical regimes, as mentioned above, are based on the same underlying anatomic, physiologic, and pathologic knowledge. Techniques of massage, bandaging and padding, exercise, and drug therapy vary between them, although some of the techniques are similar. There have been many variations of the Vodder method, particularly in Europe. All of these methods are updated and adapted continually.

The various methods (at least as they are at present) should not all be looked upon as necessarily producing the same results. Proof of their efficacy lies ultimately in their *published* results. There are also many who say that they practice "CPT" "MLD" or "lymphatic drainage" but have very dubious qualifications. Results they produce must not be taken as the equivalent of a well-trained therapist in any of the regimens. The Casley-Smith method of CPT basically uses massage techniques that differ from any of the

other methods, although, of course, some aspects are the same. The work over the watershed areas varies and is more intensive and concentrated. The exercises for CPT were developed separately and were designed specifically to mimic the sequences of the massage. The combination of physical methods with the benzopyrones was also instigated.

CONCLUSIONS

It has been proven that exercises and benzopyrones combined with CPT can play very important and statistically highly significant roles, both during the course of treatment and for further reduction after treatment. It is clear that, with postmastectomy lymphedema, the earlier the patient receives treatment, the better the prognosis, and the less the overall cost involved both in monetary terms and in quality of life. It is possible that with better diagnostic methods, e.g., further advances in lymphscintigraphy, we will be able to predict more accurately those people with limbs at risk of developing lymphedema.

However, until that time, a few prophylactic measures should be taken into account to prevent its onset.[41] These include the avoidance of any trauma, e.g., cuts or abrasions, sunburn, etc.; the overloading of the limb, e.g., carrying heavy loads; blood-pressure cuffs

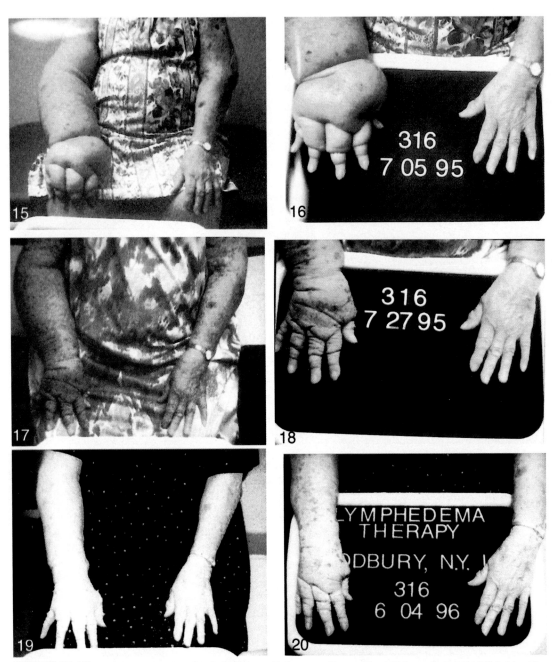

FIGURES 15–20. A large, postmastectomy lymphedemia in an elderly woman. Figures 15 and 16 (top row) show the initial state of the patient. Figures 17 and 18 (middle row) show the patient after the course of CPT, and Figures 19 and 20 (bottom row) show the patient after 1 year (courtesy of Lymphedema Therapy, NY, Boris, Lasinski, and Weindorf).

used on the limb at risk. Spotless cleanliness; keeping the skin moist and supple; immediate treatment of any infection; and, for long flights (in which the cabin pressure is lower), prophylactic compression are essential.[55] On the positive side, a person should be encouraged to lead as normal a life as possible. Prevention of lymphedema should be of foremost priority.

REFERENCES

1. Winiwater F. Das Elephantiasis "Deutsche Chirugie." Stuttgart: Enke, 1892:23.
2. Wittlinger H, Wittlinger G. Textbook of Dr. Vodder's manual lymph drainage. Vol 1, basic course, 3rd rev. Heidelberg: Haug, 1982.
3. Földi M, Kubik S. Lehrbuch der Lymphologie fur Mediziner und Physiotherapeute. Stuttgart: Fischer, 1989.

4. Földi M, Földi E. Komplexe physikalische entstauungstherapie des chronischen gliedmaben lymphnödems. *Folia Angiol* 1981;29:161–8.

5. Foldi E. Comprehensive lymphedema treatment center. *Lymphology* 1994;27:505–7.

6. Anon. The diagnosis and treatment of peripheral lymphedema. *Lymphology* 1995;28:113–7.

7. Foldi M. Treatment of lymphedema. *Lymphology* 1994;27: 1–5.

8. Casley-Smith JR, Casley-Smith JR. Modern treatment of lymphoedema, 5th ed. Malvern: The Lymphoedema Association of Australia, 1997.

9. Casley-Smith JR, Casley-Smith JR. High protein, oedema and the benzo-pyrones. Sydney: Lippincott, 1986.

10. Leduc O, Dereppe H, Hoylaerts M, Renard M, Bernard R. Hemodynamic effects of pressotherapy. In: Progress in lymphology. XII Excerpta medica, International Congress series 887. Nishi M, Uchino S, Yabuki S, editors. Amsterdam: Elsevier, 1990:431–4.

11. Casley-Smith JR, Földi M, Ryan TJ, et al. Lymphedema. Summary of the 10th International Congress of Lymphology working group discussions and recommendations. Adelaide, Australia, August 10–17, 1985. *Lymphology* 1985;18: 175–80.

12. Földi E. Prevention of dermatolymphangioadenitis by combined physiotherapy of the swollen arm after treatment for breast cancer. *Lymphology* 1996;29:48–9.

13. Okhuma M. Cellulitis seen in lymphœdema. In: Progress in Lymphology XII. Excerpta medica, International Congress series 887. Nishi M, Uchino S, Yabuki S, editors. Amsterdam: Elsevier, 1990:401–2.

14. Ohkuma M. Mycotic infection in lymphœdema. In: Progress in Lymphology XIII. Excerpta medica, International Congress series 994. Cluzan RV, Pecking AP, Lokiec FM, editors. Amsterdam; Elsevier, 1992:489–90.

15. Thiadens SRJ. A study of infection in 353 lymphedema patients and antibiotic therapy. In: Progress in Lymphology XIII. Excerpta medica, International Congress series 994. Cluzan RV, Pecking AP, Lokiec FM, editors. Amsterdam: Elsevier, 1992:477–8.

16. Olszewski WL, Jamal S, Dworczynski A, et al. Bacteriological studies of skin, tissue fluid and lymph in filianal lymphœdema. *Lymphology* 1994;27(Suppl):345–8.

17. Bedna K, Švestková S. Incidence rate of recurrent erysipelas in our lymphœedema patients. *Lymphology* 1994;27(Suppl): 519–22.

18. Pecking A, Cluzan R, Desprez-Curely JP. Indirect lymphoscintigraphy in patients with limb edema. In: *Progress in Lymphology*, Heim LR, Braf ZF, Casley-Smith JR, Dumont AE, Yoffey JM, editors. Newburgh: Immunology Research Foundation 1984:201–8.

19. Casley-Smith JR, Björlin M. Some parameters affecting the removal of œdema by massage - mechanical or manual. In: Progress in Lymphology X. Casley-Smith JR, Piller NB, editors. Adelaide: University of Adelaide Press, 1985:182–4.

20. Derdeyn A, Aslam M, Pflug JJ. Manual lymph drainage—mode of action. *Lymphology* 1994;27(Suppl):527–9.

21. Hutzschenreuter P, Bruemmer H. Influence of complex decongesting therapy on positive interstitial pressure and on lymphgiomotor activity. In: Progress in Lymphology XI. Excerpta medica, International Congress series 779. Partsch H, editor. Amsterdam: Elsevier, 1988:557–60.

22. Franzeck UK, Herrig I, Costanzo U, Hofer HO, Bollinger A. Lymphatic capillary pressure and network extension in patients with lymphœdema before and after combined physical therapy [abstract]. *Eur J Lymphol* 1995;5:149.

23. Leduc O, Bourgeois P, Leduc A. Manual lymphatic drainage: scintigraphic demonstration of its efficacy on colloidal protein reabsorption. In: Progress in Lymphology XI. Excerpta medica, International Congress series 779. Partsch H, editor. Amsterdam: Elsevier, 1988a:551–4.

24. Casley-Smith JR. Endothelial permeability. II. The passage of particles through the lymphatic endothelium of normal and injured ears. *Br J Exp Pathol* 1965;46:25–49.

25. Leduc A, Bastin R, Bourgeois P. Lymphatic reabsorption of proteins and pressotherapies. In: Progress in Lymphology XI. Excerpta medica, International Congress series 779. Partsch H, editor. Amsterdam: Elsevier, 1988b:591–2.

26. Mortimer PS. Assessment of peripheral lymph flow before and after clinical intervention. In: Progress in Lymphology XII. Excerpta medica, International Congress series 887. Nishi M, Uchino S, Yabuki S, editors. Amsterdam: Elsevier, 1990:215–22.

27. Mortimer PS, Simmonds R, Rezvani M, et al. Measurement of skin lymph flow by an isotope clearance technique: reliability, reproducibility, effect of injection dynamics and lymph flow enhancement. *J Invest Dermatol* 1990;95:677–82.

28. Casley-Smith JR. Estimation of optimal massage pressure: is this possible? *Folia Angiol* 1981;29:154–6.

29. Elissková M. Are peripheral lymphatics damaged by high pressure manual massage? *Lymphology* 1995;28:21–30.

30. Földi E. Massage and damage to lymphatics. *Lymphology* 1995;28:1–3.

31. Coleridge Smith PD, Scurr JH, Robinson KP. Optimum methods of limb compression following varicose vein surgery. *Phlebology* 1987;2:165–72.

32. Lawrence D, Kakkar VV. Graduated, static, external compression of the lower limb. *Br J Surg* 1980;67:119–21.

33. Leduc O, Klein P, Demaret P, Belgrado JP. Dymanic pressure variation under bandages with different stiffness. In: Vascular medicine, International Congress series 1018. Boccalon H, editor. Amsterdam: Elsevier, 1993:465–8.

34. Leduc O, Klein P, Demaret P, Belgrado J-P. Dynamic pressure variation under bandages with different stiffness. In: Vascular Medicine. International Congress series 1018. Boccalon H, editor. Amsterdam: Elsevier, 1993:465–8.

35. Leduc O, Peeters A, Bourgeois P. Bandages: scintigraphic demonstration of its efficacy on colloidal protein reabsorption during muscle activity. In: Progress in Lymphology XII. Excerpta medica, International Congress series 887. Nishi M, Uchino S, Yabuki S, editors. Amsterdam: Elsevier, 1990; 421–3.

36. Olszewski WL, Engeset A. Vasomotoric function of lymphatics and lymph transport in limbs during massage and with elastic support. In: Progress in Lymphology XI. Excerpta medica, International Congress series 779. Partsch H, editor. Amsterdam: Elsevier, 1988:571–5.

37. Partsch H. Verbesserte förderleistung der wadenmuskelpumpe unter kompressionstrümpfen bei Varizen und venöser Insuffizienz. *Phlebol Proktol* 1978;7:58.

38. Partsch H. Do we need firm compression stocking exerting high pressure? *Vasa* 1984;13:52–7.

39. Stemmer R, Marescaux J, Furderer C. Compression treatment of the lower extremities particularly with compression stockings. *Dermatologist* 1980;31:355–65.

40. Hohlbaum GG, Milde L, Schitz R, Weber G. The medical compression stocking. Stuttgart: Schattauer, 1989.

41. Casley-Smith JR. Exercises for patients with lymphoedema of the arm and a guide to self-massage and hydrotherapy, 5th ed. Malvern. The Lymphoedema Association of Australia, 1998.

42. Swedborg I. Effectiveness of combined methods of physiotherapy for post-mastectomy lymphœdema. *Scand J Rehab Med* 1980;12:77–85.

43. Morgan RG, Casley-Smith JR, Mason MR, Casley-Smith JR. Complex physical therapy for the lymphœdematous arm. *Br J Hand Surg* 1992;17B:437–41.

44. Casley-Smith JR, Casley-Smith JR. Lymphoedema therapy in Australia, complex physical therapy and benzo-pyrones in over 600 limbs. *Lymphology* 1994;27(Suppl):622–6.

45. Casley-Smith JR, Casley-Smith JR. Lymphoedema therapy by complex physical therapy (C.P.T.), with and without oral and topical benzo-pyrones: what should therapist and patients expect? *Lymphology* 1996;29:76–82.

46. Casley-Smith JR, Piller NB, Morgan RG. Treatment of lymphoedema of the arms and legs with 5,6 benzo-a-pyrone. *N Engl J Med* 1993a:329:1158–63.

47. Clodius L, Piller NB. The conservative treatment of post mastectomy in patients with coumarin results in a marked continuous reduction in swelling. In: Advances in Lymphology. Bartos V, Davidson JW, editors. Prague: Avicenum, 1982:471–4.

48. Cluzan R, Pecking A. Benzopyrone (Lysedem) double blind crossing over study in patients with secondary upper limb edemas. In: Progress in Lymphology XII. Excerpta Medica, International Congress series 887. Nishi M, Uchino S, Yabuki S, editors. Amsterdam: Elsevier, 1990:453–4.

49. Desprez-Curely JP, Cluzan R, Pecking A. Benzopyrones and post mastectomy lymphoedemas. Double-blind trial placebo versus sustained release coumarin with trioxyethylrutin (TER). In: Progress in Lymphology X. Casley-Smith JR, Piller NB, editors. Adelaide: University of Adelaide Press, 1985:156–8.

50. Piller NB, Clodius L. Clinical results of the effectiveness of Venalot in 103 postmastectomy lymphoedema patients: In: Advances in Lymphology. Bartos V, Davidson JW, editors. Prague: Avicenum, 1982;475–9.

51. Piller NB, Morgan RG, Casley-Smith JR. A double blind cross-over trial of O-(β-hydroxy-ethyl)-rutosides (benzo-pyrones) in the treatment of lymphoedema of the arms and legs. *Br J Plast Surg* 1988;41:20–7.

52. Boris M, Weindorf S, Lasinski B. Lymphedema reduction by noninvasive complex lymphedema therapy. *Oncology* 1994; 8:95–106.

53. Boris M, Weindorf S, Lasinski B. Persistence of lymphedema reduction after noninvasive complex lymphedema therapy. *Oncology* 1997;11:99–109.

54. Casley-Smith JR, Casley-Smith JR. The cost efficacy of various treatments for lymphoedema. *Lymphology* 1996;29:49–55.

55. Casley-Smith JR, Casley-Smith JR. Lymphœdema initiated by aircraft flights. *Aviat Space Environ Med* 1996;67:52–6.

Complete Decongestive Physiotherapy and the Lerner Lymphedema Services Academy of Lymphatic Studies (the Lerner School)

Robert Lerner, M.D.

Lerner Lymphedema Services, New York, New York.

BACKGROUND. Lymphedema is more common than most physicians realize. It is also an incurable, life long condition that has never been treated effectively in the past in our country.

METHODS. The author describes complete decongestive physiotherapy (CDP) and his contribution to making it available all across the United States. This was done by establishing a network of outpatient CDP clinics where patients can be treated effectively and a training school, the Lerner Lymphedema Services Academy of Lymphatic Studies (the Lerner School), where physicians and therapists can be trained in all facets of the lymphedema problem and where the CDP method with all of its components is taught.

RESULTS AND CONCLUSIONS. The superiority of CDP to pneumatic pumps and to surgical procedures used to treat lymphedema is discussed. A description of the Lerner School's philosophy and curriculum is included. *Cancer* 1998;83:2861–3. © 1998 American Cancer Society.

KEYWORDS: lymphedema, complete (complex) decongestive physiotherapy, Lerner Lymphedema Services Academy of Lymphatic Studies, Vodder method.

Some physicians and many patients now realize that lymphedema is tantamount to a life sentence that one receives in court, that there is no cure for lymphedema, and that the condition is progressive, i.e., it gets worse over time. Although one can never predict the rate of progression, it is certain that, without proper medical care, the condition gets worse and worse.

In the past, physicians always played down the importance of lymphedema and pointed out to generations of patients that it is very rare, that there is no effective treatment, that the patient must learn to "live with it," or even that it will get better some day or will go away. Moreover, physicians have failed to instruct patients on how to avoid lymphedema after surgery or radiation therapy and continue to grossly understate the incidence of this very serious and life-long illness.

In 1984, a National Cancer Institute publication stated that 50–70% of women who undergo axillary node surgery develop lymphedema.[1] After careful study over many years, I find these numbers to be accurate. However, I know of no surgeon or radiation therapist who, in explaining the adverse effects of a planned intervention, is apt to cite those figures. Many avoid mentioning lymphedema at all.

Even patients undergoing lumpectomy, limited axillary dissection, and radiation therapy—the so-called conservative procedure— develop lymphedema in the upper extremity, in the adjacent body

Presented at the American Cancer Society Lymphedema Workshop, New York, New York, February 20–22, 1998.

Dr. Lerner is affiliated with the Memorial Sloan-Kettering Cancer Center, New York, New York.

Address for reprints: Robert Lerner, M.D., Lerner Lymphedema Services, P.C., 245 East 63rd Street, Suite 106. New York, NY 10021.

Received July 2, 1998; accepted August 20, 1998.

quadrant, and often in the radiated breast with great frequency. The incidence of lymphedema after breast conservation surgery was the same or higher than it was after radical or modified radical mastectomy, because axillary radiation and axillary dissection act synergistically in producing lymphedema.[2]

Over the past 10–15 years, surgeons have been excising fewer and fewer nodes in an effort to decrease the lymphedema problem. In the last 3–4 years, there has been a great effort to learn and to employ the sentinel node biopsy technique in breast carcinoma patients, a procedure borrowed from melanoma surgery.

Some surgeons have totally eliminated axillary dissection for various kinds of breast carcinoma and in certain categories of patients. It is reasonable to predict that axillary dissection for breast carcinoma definitely is on the way out and will be gone before long. Certainly, there ought to be a less invasive and more accurate method of diagnosing positive axillary lymph nodes.

Lymphedema Therapies

At the present time, there are only three common lymphedema treatments: pneumatic pumps, surgical procedures, and complete decongestive physiotherapy (CDP). Our school, the Lerner Lymphedema Services Academy of Lymphatic Studies (The Lerner School), is strongly opposed to the use of pneumatic pumps for a variety of reasons: 1) The pumps do not evacuate fluid from the ipsilateral body quadrant, which is also congested in extremity lymphedema. 2) The pumps "milk" excess interstitial fluid from the upper or lower extremity to the shoulder, the lower abdomen, the pelvis. 3) In lower extremity lymphedema, pumping can cause swelling of the external genitalia. 4) Pumps have no value in Stage II or Stage III lymphedema because of the presence of scar and fibrous tissue. 5) Pumps, like blood pressure cuffs, may traumatize residual, still functioning lymph vessels. 6) Unless the patient wraps the limb following each pumping session, edema fluid soon returns. 7) Over time, the lymphedema worsens in patients who use pneumatic pumps.

Patients who use pneumatic pumps sooner or later realize the pump's lack of efficacy and stop using it. In a recent survey done by the Greater Boston Lymphedema Support Group,[3] it was shown that, of 56 members who had been using a pneumatic pump, 43 (78%) no longer used it. The reason most frequently given for discontinuing the pump was that it was doing nothing, it was not helping, or it caused various undesirable side effects, such as swelling in an adjacent area, pain, or soreness.

These results underscore our own patient data,[4] which showed that 96 of 149 upper extremity patients and 100 of 150 lower extremity patients had already given up the pneumatic pump when they came for initial consultation at our center. The reasons they gave for abandoning pump therapy were lack of any beneficial effect, the swollen limb was getting worse, the benefit was too transitory, or the swelling in an adjacent body area had become more noticeable. Four lower extremity patients gave up the pump because pumping caused abdominal fluid accumulation that led to the fallacious diagnosis of pelvic tumor and, in three patients, to unnecessary exploratory laparotomy.

Surgical therapies for lymphedema have been available for the past century. Procedures of all types have been recommended, most of which bear the name of the innovator, e.g., Kondoleon,[5] Homans,[6] Thompson,[7] Charles,[8] Goldsmith,[9] Standard,[10] etc. Most of them have been abandoned because of poor results or serious morbidity/mortality figures. Some plastic surgeons continue to practice some of the resectional procedures just mentioned, and several centers continue to use one of the numerous microsurgical procedures available: lymphovenous anastomosis,[11] lymph vessel transplantation,[12] or autologous small vein transplantation.[13] We continue to await the long term results of these latter procedures. In the meantime, we at the Lerner School recommend surgery only for chylous reflux, for exision of fistulous tracts associated with intestinal lymphangiectasia, and, occasionally, to remove redundant, loose skin folds that sometimes remain after a course of CDP therapy.

The third method of treating lymphedema is generally called complex or complete decongestive physiotherapy (CDP). Some people refer to this procedure as CDT, CDPT, or combined physiotherapy. Whenever I am invited to speak, I appeal to all who work in the field of lymphology to use the same term, just so that we all know what we are talking about. I recommend CDP, because it is the original name, the name by which everyone recognizes the two-phase, noninvasive procedure: physicians, physiotherapists, insurance companies, Medicare, etc.

The Lerner School

At the Lerner School, we teach everything there is to know about the CDP method. Although we are not the Vodder School, our instructors are Vodder manual lymph drainage (MLD)/CDP-certified instructors, and we teach the Vodder method of MLD as modified and improved by the Foldi School.

We have no desire to compete with courses given by others over a weekend or even over a 5-day period. Nor are we interested in therapists who attempt to train themselves by watching a videotape or two over any period of time.

The Lerner School is the largest school of its kind in the United States at present. Courses are given six to eight times a year; most are given either in Princeton, New Jersey, or in Fort Lauderdale, Florida. Students attending these courses spend some of their training time at our nearby clinics for first-hand observation of therapy in progress, measuring and fitting of support garments, and one-on-one interaction with physicians who specialize in lymphedema therapy.

Each course is comprised of 135 60-minute hours of instruction given over a 14-day period. Students (physicians, physical therapists, occupational therapists, registered nurses, and massage therapists) learn the anatomy, physiology, and pathophysiology of the lymphatic system; the laws governing the formation and transportation of lymph fluid; Vodder's MLD techniques; lymphedema bandaging techniques; measuring and fitting of support garments; complications of lymphedema; skin and nail care; diet and nutrition in lymphedema; remedial exercises, etc.

When we started our training program, MLD and CDP were unknown in the United States. We were concerned primarily at that time with preparing therapists to work in our own lymphedema clinic in New York and, somewhat later, in our Princeton clinic as well.

We felt that it was easier to train American therapists in the United States and in English than to bring trained therapists from Europe or to send Americans overseas for their training. We believe it is essential to include massage therapists in our student body, because experience has shown that this group is the most likely to give up all other professional activities and devote themselves exclusively to treating lymphedema patients. We also believe very strongly that MLD/CDP therapists must work under the direct supervision of physicians who have competence and expertise in lymphedema.

The Lerner School has become the largest and most successful MLD/CDP school in the United States. I have been the director of the school since its inception; the two principal instructors are certified Vodder MLD/CDP therapists and certified Vodder MLD/CDP instructors, each having many years of experience in treating lymphedema patients and in training therapists.

Because of our efforts, our clinics in New York, New Jersey, Massachusetts, and Florida have been able to amass the most extensive American experience treating lymphedema patients since we started using the CDP method in 1989. Thus far, we have treated more than 4000 patients with all varieties and stages of lymphedema: extremity, head and neck, genital, pure and combined forms, etc. We have also been able to train therapists for our own network of clinics and for many of the most prestigious American hospitals: the Mayo Clinic, Stanford University, Massachusetts General Hospital, Memorial Sloan-Kettering Cancer Center, Brigham and Women's Hospital, the Dana Farber Cancer Center, etc.

In all of our efforts to establish CDP as the treatment of choice for lymphedema in the United States, we recognize the pioneering work of Professor M. Foldi, who did so much to popularize the method and who elucidated so eloquently the physiology and pathophysiology of lymphedema. By employing his CDP method, we have been given a treatment modality that achieves a greater than 80% long term success rate without morbidity or mortality and without disfigurement of any kind. We have been able to do all of this for a reasonable cost, and, by transferring the future care of the lymphedema patient away from the doctor/hospital setting, we have produced a very cost effective method of caring for this long term, chronic disease.

REFERENCES

1. National Cancer Institute. The breast cancer digest. 2nd ed. Bethesda, MD: Office of Cancer Communications, National Cancer Institute, 1984:78.
2. Petrek JA, Lerner R. Lymphedema. In: Diseases of the Breast. Philadelphia: Lippincott-Raven, 1996:896–903.
3. Lynnworth, M. Greater Boston Lymphedema Support Group Pump Survey. In: *Newslett Natl Lymphedema Network* 1988;10:6–7.
4. Ko DSC, Lerner R, Klose G, Cosimi AB. Effective treatment of lymphedema of the extremities, Presentation to the New England Surgical Society Annual Meeting, Saratoga Springs, NY: September 20, 1997.
5. Kondoleon E. Die chirurgische Behandlung der Lymphableitung. *Munch Med Wochschr* 1912;59:2726–9.
6. Homans J. Treatment of elephantiasis of the legs. *N Engl J Med* 1936;215:1099.
7. Thompson N. The surgical treatment of postmastectomy lymphedema of the upper limb. *Scand J Plast Reconstr Surg* 1969;3:56–60.
8. Dumanian GA, Futrell JW. The Charles Procedure: misquoted and misunderstood since 1950. *Plast Reconstr Surg* 1996;98:1258–63.
9. Goldsmith HS. Long-term evaluation of omental transposition for chronic lymphedema. *Ann Surg* 1974;180:847–9.
10. Standard S. Lymphedema of the arm following radical mastectomy for carcinoma of the breast; new operation for its control. *Ann Surg* 1942;116:816–20.
11. Degni M. New microsurgical technique of lymphaticovenous anastomosis for treatment of lymphedema. *Lymphology* 1981;14:61–3.
12. Baumeister RGH. Clinical results of autologous lymphatic grafts in the treatment of lymphedemas. In: Lymphology XI. Partsch H, editor. Amsterdam: Elsevier Science Publishers BV, 1988:419–20.
13. Campisi C. Use of autologous interposition vein graft in management of lymphedema. *Lymphology* 1991;24:71–6.

Current Status of Education and Treatment Resources for Lymphedema

Saskia R. J. Thiadens, R.N.

National Lymphedema Network, Inc., San Francisco, California.

BACKGROUND. Secondary lymphedema (LE) resulting from breast cancer surgery has continued to be an ignored medical diagnosis in U.S. medicine. Subsequently, the majority of women/men undergoing axillary lymph node dissection have not received education in pre- or postoperative LE prevention, causing hundreds of thousands of patients to develop LE. As a result of this ignorance, once the LE develops, these patients receive no or harmful treatment.

METHODS. Over the last decade, the National Lymphedema Network (NLN) has created awareness in the medical community, among patients, and in the general public through information dissemination, educational materials, a national conference, and the activism of patients and a small group of concerned professionals. Complete decongestive physiotherapy (CDP), which includes manual lymph drainage, is a successful treatment for LE that has now been introduced.

RESULTS. Slowly, the U.S. medical community is beginning to recognize and support this condition and its treatment, and secondary LE has now become an acceptable diagnosis (ICD9-457.0). Subsequently, due to patient and medical activism and the work of the NLN, Medicare now covers 2 weeks of CDP treatment (in Florida), and two landmark bills (AB-12 and S-609) that will cover LE treatment for postbreast carcinoma patients are currently pending (as of February 22, 1998).

CONCLUSIONS. In the last decade, the NLN has developed a strong foundation of knowledge and has planted LE on the medical map in the United States. With collaboration between the NLN and all breast carcinoma groups and LE specialists, it is hoped that lymphology will become a standard course of study in medical schools across the country and that LE will become a household word, with proper treatment available for postbreast carcinoma LE patients in the United States. *Cancer* **1998;83:2864–8.** © *1998 American Cancer Society.*

KEYWORDS: complete decongestive physiotherapy, manual lymph drainage, National Lymphedema Network, secondary lymphedema.

Lymphology is essentially an overlooked field in medical schools in the United States, and, because of this and other important factors, medical professionals have been exposed inadequately to this poor step child of U.S. medicine. As the breast carcinoma rate continues to increase in the United States, so too does the incidence of upper extremity lymphedema among both women and men who have undergone modified radical mastectomies, lumpectomies, or simple mastectomies. The question is, why is such an important area of study and treatment ignored? Is this because lymphedema is considered a chronic, incurable condition, or is it a lack of knowledge and interest on the part of physicians who are the first line of contract for breast carcinoma patients? Because breast carcinoma affects mostly women, is this a factor in the level of attention that secondary lymphedema has received? These are questions we all need to con-

Presented at the American Cancer Society Lymphedema Workshop, New York, New York, February 20–22, 1998.

The author gratefully acknowledges Mitchelle Tanner, editor.

Address for reprints: Saskia R.J. Thiadens, R.N., National Lymphedema Network, Inc., 2211 Post Street, Suite 404, San Francisco, CA 94115-3417.

Received July 2, 1998; accepted August 20, 1998.

sider in order to move forward. Certainly, one of the main reasons patients continue to be told that "nothing can be done" is that most professionals in the medical community are not aware of the effective, safe treatments currently available for patients following breast carcinoma surgery.

Over the past decade, there has been a marked increase in the scope and availability of treatment options for lymphedema. This is due in great part to a wave of activism by patients who have been angered by the lack of information and unavailability of appropriate treatment. These patients, in turn, have motivated their health care providers to become more involved in and educated about lymphedema. Today, a handful of dedicated professionals are leading the way toward eventual standardization of treatment and training in the United States.

Ignorance and Resistance within the Medical Community

Despite continuing ignorance and resistance within much of the medical community, secondary lymphedema related to breast carcinoma has become a recognized and acceptable medical diagnosis categorized under the code ICD9-457.0. However, even when it is diagnosed, thousands of lymphedema patients encounter physicians who are unaware of recent developments in lymphedema treatment. Many still rely on outdated methods that were popular 30–40 years ago, such as the use of diuretics (ineffective and potentially harmful to the patient) and elevation (unrealistic). An example of the negative effects of outdated treatment on both patient care and efficient use of medical coverage is the continuing prescription of pumps. These are often delivered with no patient orientation or follow-up and, in some cases, actually worsen the condition irreversibly. Though pumps do have a place in patient treatment programs, especially in the early stages, it is crucial that they be used in conjunction with complimentary modalities (such as manual lymph drainage [MLD] and compression bandaging).

Consequences of Ignorance

When a condition such as lymphedema (and the lymphatic system in general) continues to be ignored, it impacts both patients and health care professionals; patients often become frightened and lose respect for their providers, with many experiencing severe complications and often devastating life and psychological changes—such as loss of employment, divorce, functional limitations, and subsequent loss of independence—all of which could be avoided. However, not only are the patients impacted, but a crucial piece of the medical puzzle is lost when an entire anatomical system is not addressed. Ignorance and lack of interest

in lymphology does a disservice to us all, because the data and information that can be gained from research into this field will impact the entire body of medical knowledge in the United States.

Lymphedema Awareness and Education

In 1987, I opened the first lymphedema clinic in the United States. Much of what I encountered at that time I continue to see today, although the climate and level of participation is slowly beginning to change. At that time, patients were self-referred, because no physicians knew about treatment, and I began to hear the first wave of repeating horror stories. The most common response that patients received was "do not worry about it, it will go away," or "you will just have to learn to live with it." Of course, once the patient continued on without treatment or education, multiple physical and psychological complications ensued. Treatments that *were* prescribed included elevating the arm(s) by securing it to an IV or other type of pole while sleeping, using heating pads, securing wide rubber bands at intervals up the arm, wrapping with ace bandages, and using diuretics long term in high doses. Of course, diuretics at this level can be extremely harmful and can cause electrolyte imbalances, endangering the kidneys and risking heart failure. I believe that the other modalities speak for themselves.

I became aware of the dire need for education, and, after discovering treatment modalities used in Europe for the past 3 decades, in 1988, I founded the National Lymphedema Network (NLN). The goals of the NLN have been and continue to be the education of lymphedema patients and health care professionals, creating awareness about the condition within the general public, and empowering patients to care for themselves, subsequently educating their medical teams.

However, it has taken many years to get the medical community to listen and to identify this often very serious and disabling condition. We are only now just scratching the surface. Over the years, the NLN has disseminated information to hundreds of thousands of health care professionals, patients, family members, and the general public, working hard to create awareness through many avenues. These include information packets, a quarterly newsletter, treatment referrals and guidance, a biennial conference, and, more recently, an extensive online educational website.

Today, women who are diagnosed with breast carcinoma are encountering a growing number of health care professionals, facilities, and breast carcinoma organizations who are familiar with lymphedema, preventive methods, and the NLN (including the American Cancer Society, Y-Me, the National Alliance

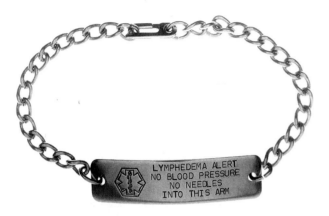

FIGURE 1. The lymphedema alert bracelet.

of Breast Cancer Organizations, Susan Komen, the National Breast Cancer Coalition, and support groups across the country). A major goal of the NLN is to work closely with these and other breast carcinoma organizations across the country, combining all of our knowledge and resources to educate and support every patient diagnosed with breast carcinoma or lymphedema. By empowering patients with information, we have learned that not only are they better able to care for themselves and improve their quality of life, but many have become key players in motivating health care professionals and hospitals to set up lymphedema treatment centers across the country; some patients have gone so far as to raise the funds themselves to set up the facility.

In early January of this year, an especially driven breast carcinoma and lymphedema patient, Karin Douglas, in partnership with the NLN, created the first lymphedema alert bracelet (Fig. 1). This bracelet is designed to protect patients at risk of or who have already developed lymphedema from receiving chemotherapy, blood pressures, or needle injections into their affected arm(s). In addition, it is hoped that they will provide education about lymphedema to health care professionals and medical teams who care for these patients.

Treatment Resources and Support Groups

Because the management of lymphedema is still inconsistent, and the atmosphere is chaotic, it is often difficult for patients and professionals alike to know where and how to look for treatment options and what exactly to ask for. It is amazing to note that, in Europe, for decades, there have been entire hospitals established just for the treatment of lymphedema and related conditions. In these facilities, patients undergo 4 full weeks of inpatient therapy. Because of the current structure of the medical and insurance industries here

in the United States, as well as a shortage of treatment centers and professionals across the country, U.S. practitioners must attempt to accomplish the same results in only 1 or 2 weeks.

At present, the NLN has 69 affiliated treatment centers, 29 certified therapists, and over 100 lymphedema support groups as well as established diagnostic centers where ongoing research is conducted (Fig. 2). It is a start. However, every year we receive more than 30,000 calls from patients and health care professionals seeking referrals and answers to their many questions. Because the number of clinics providing safe, effective care for lymphedema is limited, patients often have to travel considerable distances to receive treatment, often outside of their home state or across the country. For this reason, it is very important to investigate referrals before the patient makes an appointment to be sure that the care provided meets their medical as well as financial needs. In fact, there have been a few cases in which patients secured loans or sold property to pay for care, only to find that the care they received actually worsened their condition. Because of this and similar problems, it is vital that we work together for the common cause of quality treatment for all patients and move toward a consensus and standardization of basic treatment identified by the American Medical Association.

Some Questions to Ask when Contacting a Lymphedema Treatment Center

The following questions are recommended to patients seeking treatment. This list of questions also offers guidance to those facilities interested in setting up a lymphedema program.

1. Do you provide a complete decongestive physiotherapy (CDP) program?
2. Do you provide bandaging, compression sleeves, or any other nonmechanical compression devices?
3. Does your staff consist of certified fitters for compression garments?
4. Do you provide education in: exercises, skin care, diet, nutritional supplements, and complimentary holistic therapies?
5. What kind of results should I expect, and will I be taught how to maintain the reduction through self-massage and/or self-bandaging as well as partner participation?
6. Will I need a referral or prescription from my doctor for the treatment?
7. What are the program options (5-day, 10-day, or 21-day intensives)? Are longer programs available if I need them?

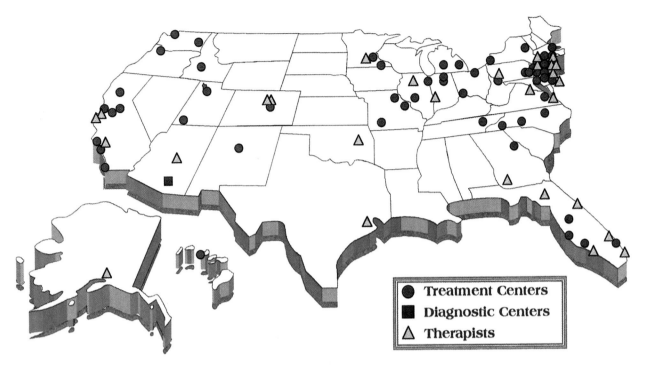

FIGURE 2. National Lymphedema Network-affiliated treatment centers, diagnostic centers, and certified therapists.

8. What is the cost of the program(s), and are the supplies included in the cost?

9. Will there be assistance available in emergency situations on weekends and/or evenings?

10. Are your patients required to pay up front out of pocket, or will your office bill insurance?

11. What kind of training/experience in lymphedema treatment does your clinical director and on-staff therapists have?

12. May I contact a patient with a condition similar to mine who has been treated by your facility?

13. Does your facility offer a support group?[1]

Insurance Issues

Due to lack of knowledge and recognition of effective treatment for lymphedema, obtaining insurance reimbursement has been an uphill battle. In the present climate of managed care, too many patients are denied treatment. Often, insurance companies claim that this type of therapy is "hocus pocus" and that legitimate clinical data are needed. Over the last decade, and as a result of increased interest, there is noticeable improvement in the reimbursement rates. There is a growing realization among insurance providers that, if it is left untreated, then lymphedema will lead ultimately to serious and expensive complications. Insurance coverage is also highly dependent on the location of the patient; in which state they are being treated. In October, 1997, CDP therapy was ac-

cepted as a covered treatment by Florida Medicare when prescribed as "medically necessary." The CDP must be performed by a "health care professional who has received specialized training in this treatment," and the therapy must be provided either by or under the direct personal supervision of the physician or an independently practicing physical therapist. The goal of this therapy is not to achieve maximum reduction but, ultimately, to transfer the responsibility of the care from the clinic, hospital, or doctor to home care by the patient, patient's family, or care giver. Hopefully, commercial insurance carriers who, until now, may have used the Medicare position as a rationale for refusing coverage will now begin to cover CDP as well.[2]

Legislation

In April, 1997, two landmark bills were introduced, one in California (AB-12) and one on Capitol Hill (S-609). The first bill, AB-12, a California Assembly bill, addresses a number of issues that will impact mastectomy patients in California, including coverage of "prosthetic devices or reconstructive surgery, including devices or surgery to restore and achieve symmetry for the patient," and all complications from a mastectomy, "*including lymphedema.*"

The second bill, S-609, a U.S. Senate bill cited as *The Reconstructive Breast Surgery Benefits Act of 1997,* was presented by Senator Edward Kennedy on April

17, 1997. This bill, if passed, will "amend the Public Health Service Act and Employee Retirement Income Security Act of 1974 to require that group and individual health insurance coverage and group health plans provide coverage for reconstructive breast surgery if they provide coverage for mastectomies," and that prostheses "used to establish symmetry" be covered as well as "*complications of mastectomy including lymphedema.*" These bills should be addressed in March or April of this year and, if passed, will be a milestone in a decade of work on the part of the NLN and practitioners and patients across the country.

Need for Research

Recently, a promising medical/scientific research project was launched by the NLN. Participating members from around the country—including geneticists, scientists, clinicians, and patient families—have begun brainstorming and identifying specific needs in lymphedema research, covering issues related to both primary and secondary lymphedema. Currently, the group is actively communicating with the National Institutes of Health (NIH), and two patient families will be meeting with the NIH on March 26. The goal is to organize a collaborative think-tank workshop (supported by the NIH) to identify areas of needed research and possible funding sources, including, among other things, a possible link between primary lymphedema and its relation to secondary lymphedema (i.e., does one form predispose a patient to the other?).

CONCLUSION

Obviously, there is an ongoing, pressing need for research into all aspects of the lymphatic system, from basic anatomy and physiology, to more complex vascular and lymphatic anomalies. The knowledge gained from this research then needs to be incorporated into the standard educational curriculum of all medical schools in the United States to produce graduates with a strong understanding of the lymphatic system and related conditions, such as lymphedema.

Every day, I have to ask the question: why has this area of medicine been ignored for so many years? Why are the majority of professionals currently in practice unable to identify lymphedema and often misdiagnose it? In the last 2 decades, a tremendous amount of energy and research funding has gone into the field of breast carcinoma; however, lymphedema, one form of which is related directly to breast carcinoma, has received little or not attention. We must remember that, if there was no breast carcinoma, then we would no longer see related secondary lymphedema. Thus, it is crucial that the NLN, all breast cancer organizations, and lymphedema specialists across the country work together to educate, to inform, and to support research into this long neglected condition. I look forward to the day when the words "nothing can be done for you, you just have to learn to live with it" are never heard again; when all professionals and patients are educated about lymphedema, prevention, and treatment.

REFERENCES

1. Rovig J, Miller M, Thiadens S. Suggested guidelines: questions to ask when contacting a lymphedema treatment center [special circular]. *NLN Newsletter* 1995.
2. Schuch WJ. CDP to be covered by medicare. *NLN Newsletter* 1997:8.

American Cancer Society Lymphedema Workshop

Supplement to Cancer

Lymphedema Management Training for Physical Therapy Students in the United States

Elizabeth Augustine, M.S., P.T.[1]
Matthew Corn, B.S., P.T.[2]
Jerome Danoff, Ph.D., P.T.[3]

[1] Physical Therapy Section, Rehabilitation Medicine Department, National Institutes of Health, Bethesda, Maryland.

[2] P.T. Resources, Telluride, Colorado.

[3] Department of Physical Therapy, Howard University, Washington, D.C.

Presented at the American Cancer Society Lymphedema Workshop, New York, New York, February 20–22, 1998.

The authors thank Dr. Maggie Rinehart-Ayers, Dr. Cindy Pfalzer, Bonnie Lasinski, DeCourcy Squire, and Linda Miller for critiquing the survey instrument. Special thanks are extended to Dr. Lynn Gerber for her support, to Charles McGarvey for his insights and direction throughout the study, and to Dana Strickland for her secretarial support.

Elizabeth Augustine is a Senior Staff Physical Therapist in the Physical Therapy Section of the Rehabilitation Medicine Department, National Institutes of Health.

Matthew Corn was a physical therapy student intern from the University of Hartford, Connecticut, when this study was conducted.

Jerome Danoff is an Associate Professor in the Department of Physical Therapy at Howard University and is a Research Consultant to the Rehabilitation Medicine Department at the National Institutes of Health.

Address for reprints: Elizabeth Augustine, M.S., P.T., Physical Therapy Section, Rehabilitation Medicine Department, National Institutes of Health, Building 10, Room 6s235, Bethesda, MD 20892.

The opinions expressed herein reflect the views of the authors and not those of the National Institutes or the U.S. Public Health Service.

Received July 2, 1998; accepted August 20, 1998.

BACKGROUND. The objective of this study was to determine to what extent accredited physical therapy programs in the United States were presenting the principles of lymphedema management and whether regional differences existed.
METHODS. States were grouped into four geographic regions: Northeast, South, Midwest, and West. From mid-June to mid-July, 1997, 63 of 148 (42.6%) accredited physical therapy (PT) programs in the United States completed and returned the questionnaires. Participants received a cover letter, consent form, and lymphedema survey by e-mail, facsimile, or regular post. The lymphedema survey covered a wide variety of issues relating to five areas: 1) general and 2) specific anatomy and physiology of the lymphatic system, 3) pathogenesis of lymphedema, 4) traditional (compression pumps/garments), and 5) innovative (European/Australian) treatment techniques for lymphedema. "Yes" responses indicated that specific information was included in the curriculum. Frequency of yes responses for each of the five areas were counted and converted into percentages. Regional responses were compared with the total combined responses with a modified binomial technique.
RESULTS. PT programs in the United States were providing 89% of our designated content in the general anatomy and physiology of the lymphatic system, 73% in the pathogenesis of lymphedema, 65% in traditional treatment techniques, 48% in innovative treatment techniques, and 42% in the specific anatomy and physiology of the lymphatic system. No individual region differed significantly ($P > 0.05$) from the combined results.
CONCLUSIONS. The participating PT programs appeared to be providing instruction in general anatomy and physiology of the lymphatic system, pathogenesis of lymphedema, and traditional treatment techniques. However, far less instruction on the specific anatomy and physiology of the lymphatic system and innovative treatment techniques is offered. We believe that PT students would benefit with more curricular content in these latter two categories in order to acquire the knowledge and skills to combat the devastating effects of lymphedema. *Cancer* **1998;83:2869–73.** © *1998 American Cancer Society.*

KEYWORDS: lymphedema, education, survey, physical therapy, modalities.

Lymphedema is a high-protein edema caused by a defect in the lymphatic transport capacity.[1] Lymphedema can be divided into two classifications: primary (idiopathic) and secondary (acquired). Primary lymphedema can be subdivided further into three types: congenital, praecox, and tarda. Infestation of the lymphatic system by nematodes (i.e., Wuchereria bancrofti, Brugia malayi) is the world's leading cause of secondary lymphedema.[2] In developed nations like the United States, lymphedema is a potential complication following surgical and/or radiation therapy for carcinoma.[2] It is estimated that millions of Americans suffer from lymphedema.[3,4] Once a person develops lymphedema, there is no cure for it. Consequently, the person must manage the lymphedema daily for the rest of his or her life. Lymphedema worsens if it is left untreated.

Physical impairments caused by lymphedema include pain, increased limb girth, increased limb volume, decreased strength, decreased range of motion, and impaired function. There is also a psychosocial morbidity associated with lymphedema that can include social isolation, depression, and even suicidal ideation.[5] Once a person is diagnosed with lymphedema, what happens next? Some people are told that they have to learn to live with it.[5] Others are referred to a compression pump vendor to rent or purchase a pump for home use. Many are referred to physical therapy for treatment.

The modes of lymphedema treatment may vary according to the type of education and training the physical therapist has received. Traditionally, in the United States, physical therapy treatment has included the use of compression pumps followed by fitting of compression garments. European and Australian therapists, however, favor a series of innovative treatment techniques often referred to as complex physical therapy (CPT).[1,6] CPT is used to facilitate the opening of collateral lymphatic vessels to increase drainage from obstructed areas into normal lymphotomes.[3] The components of CPT are skin care, manual lymph drainage, compression bandaging, exercises, and, finally, the fitting of a compression garment for maintenance.[1] The use of multiple modalities for the treatment of lymphedema is not new to the United States. In the 1950s and 1960s, the Mayo Clinic reported using an approach similar to CPT for lymphedema management.[7,8] In 1995, the International Society of Lymphology also recommended multiple modalities for the treatment of lymphedema.[9] Although many studies have looked at the diagnosis and treatment of the lymphedematous patient, little evidence exists whether the entry-level physical therapist possesses the essential knowledge to recognize and treat lymphedema effectively by using newer techniques.

Purpose

We examined the nature and scope of information provided to entry-level physical therapy students enrolled in accredited programs in the United States. Survey questions were grouped into five areas:

1) basic knowledge of the lymphatic system
2) specific knowledge of the lymphatic system
3) pathogenesis of lymphedema
4) traditional treatment techniques for lymphedema

5) innovative treatment techniques for lymphedema.

Theoretical curricular content on lymphedema management between programs was also examined for regional differences. This research proposal was reviewed and approved by the Research Review Committee of the Rehabilitation Medicine Department, Clinical Center, National Institutes of Health.

Subjects

To comply with the Federal Paper Reduction Act (1984), all accredited physical therapy programs were contacted initially by telephone.[10] If the response was affirmative to participate, then the director was asked to specify the form in which he or she would prefer to receive the questionnaire: e-mail, facsimile, or regular post. All participants received a cover letter stating the mission of the survey, a consent form, and a lymphedema questionnaire. Participants were asked to return the consent form and questionnaire within 2 weeks. For data analysis, U.S. physical therapy programs were divided into four geographical regions: northeast (NE), south (S), midwest (MW), and west (W).

Instrumentation

A 33-item, yes-or-no questionnaire was developed around theoretical curricular content on lymphedema management presented in U.S. physical therapy programs (Appendix A). The questions fell into five categories:

1) general anatomy and physiology of the lymphatic system
2) specific anatomy and physiology of the lymphatic system
3) pathogenesis of lymphedema
4) traditional treatment techniques for lymphedema
5) innovative treatment techniques (CPT) for lymphedema.

Respondents could write additional comments in the survey's margin to communicate a better understanding of that particular physical therapy program.

Before distribution, the survey was reviewed by clinical and academic experts for clarity and content validity. Revisions included adding more questions and rewording some items for clarity. The survey was then returned to the same experts for a second review, and a few more minor changes were made.

Data Analysis

All survey questions had two possible responses: "yes" or "no" (a binomial system). Yes responses indicated that specific information was included in the curriculum. The five-category breakdown of the question-

TABLE 1
Percentage of Specific Curricular Content on Lymphedema Management Presented in United States Physical Therapy Programs

Area	General anatomy and physiology (%)	Specific anatomy and physiology (%)	Pathogenesis (%)	Traditional techniques (%)	Innovative techniques (%)
Northeast	91	37	64	60	45
South	86	47	76	63	53
Midwest	91	44	79	71	48
West	91	33	69	70	43
Combined	89	42	73	65	48

naire was not supplied to the survey participants. Using a Power Macintosh 7200/90 computer (Apple Computers, Inc., Cupertino, CA) and Microsoft Excel version 5.0 software (Microsoft, Inc., Redmond, WA), the frequencies of these responses were recorded for each question and categorized by topics and regions. The percentage of yes responses within each category was determined. This total was interpreted as the percentage of information identified in our survey regarding the theoretical curricular content on lymphedema management being taught in the responding physical therapy programs for that particular category. Total percentages for each of the five categories were broken down by geographic region to check for regional differences.

Combined data from all regions were used to establish binomial distributions for each of the five categories. Then, the mean for each distribution is equal to the number in sample $\times$ probability (percentage) of yes responses (NP), and the standard deviation is the square root of NPQ (where Q is the probability [percentage] of no responses; also Q $= 1 - $ P). This distribution is a normal curve approximation of the binomial distribution, which is appropriate when n > 20, and allows statistical testing with Z tables.[11] The five distributions representing the entire country were used to calculate "expected values" for each of the regions that we were able to compare with each region's "observed values" by using Z tests. These tests would then show whether any individual region differed from the pattern of the entire country.

Results

During June and July, 1997, 63 of 148 (42.6%) U.S. accredited physical therapy programs completed and returned the consent forms and questionnaires. Percentages of programs in each region that participated in the survey were as follows: 33.3% NE region, 52.3% S region, 38.5% MW region, and 50% W region. Table 1 summaries regional responses to the five areas of curricular content on lymphedema amanagement.

Physical therapy programs reported that they provided 89% of our designated content in general anatomy and physiology of the lymphatic system, 42% of specific anatomy and physiology of the lymphatic system, 73% of pathogenesis of lymphedema; 65% in traditional treatment techniques, and 48% of innovative treatment techniques. No individual region differed significantly (binomial test; $P > 0.05$) from the combined results (Fig. 1). The most common remark written in the margins of the survey referred to the lack of time in the curriculum to cover more material on lymphedema management.

Discussion

According to this survey, responding physical therapy programs appeared to be providing instruction in general anatomy and physiology of the lymphatic system, pathogenesis of lymphedema, and traditional treatment techniques. However, far less instruction was reported in areas of specific anatomy and physiology of the lymphatic system and innovative treatment techniques. Also, no significant regional differences were seen in curricular content on lymphedema management ($P > 0.05$).

We questioned why the numbers of yes responses to the lymphedema questions related to the specific anatomy and physiology of the lymphatic system and innovative treatment techniques were so much lower than those of other categories of questions. We believe it is because these two categories are related: To apply many of the innovative treatment techniques successfully, one must possess knowledge of the specific anatomy and physiology of the lymphatic system.

A major obstacle in educating U.S. physical therapy students on the management of lymphedema appears to be the lack of time in the curriculum dedicated to this topic. Also, there are few textbooks published in the United States on lymphedema management. Nevertheless, innovative clinical treatment techniques, such as CPT, are currently being taught in U.S. physical therapy programs. Additional emphasis on the specifics of the lymphatic system could result

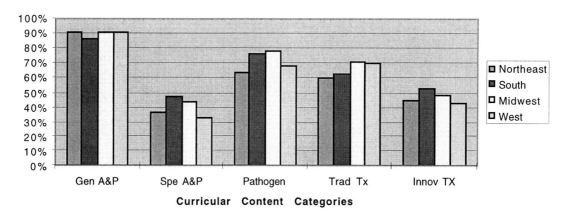

FIGURE 1. Regional distribution of curricular content on lymphedema management.

in development of better approaches and greater skills in the treatment of this condition.

Limitations

A major limiting factor in this study may have been the time of administration. Initial contact was made with the universities at the end of the academic year (June). Many faculty members were preparing for examinations, were on vacation, or had only 9–10 month appointments. This timing may have lowered the response rate. Either earlier contact or allowing a longer grace period for responses could have improved the response rate.

This survey did not ask faculty members where they obtained their training in lymphedema management, nor did it ask which references they used when developing that portion of the course. This information might have been useful for differentiating course content among programs. Consequently, this study cannot report on the continuity, quality, or depth of information provided to physical therapy students.

CONCLUSIONS

Lymphedema is a progressive condition that can have profound adverse effects on the patient's quality of life. The results of this nationwide survey confirm that physical therapy programs are supplying a large amount of information on general anatomy and physiology of the lymphatic system, pathogenesis of lymphedema, and traditional treatment techniques involved with lymphedema management. Less instruction is given on the specific anatomy and physiology of the lymphatic system and on innovative treatment techniques. We saw no significant differences among the four regions of the United States in the curricular content on lymphedema management in various physical therapy programs surveyed. Informa-tion on specific anatomy and physiology of the lymphatic system and on innovative treatment techniques not only is appropriate but is essential for providing the best possible treatment. Entry-level physical therapists must possess enough knowledge to make the right clinical decisions when choosing among various treatment options. We hope that these findings will fuel future studies on how to provide the clinician with all of the skills necessary to combat the devastating effects of lymphedema.

REFERENCES

1. Casley-Smith JR. Modern treatment of lymphoedema. *Mod Med Austr* 1992;35(5):70–83.
2. Witte MH, Witte CL, Mortimer PS, Jamal S. Lymphedema in the developing and developed world: contrasts and prospects. *Lymphology* 1988;21:242–3.
3. Boris M, Weindorf S, Lasinski B, Boris G. Lymphedema reduction by noninvasive complex lymphedema therapy. *Oncology* 1994;8:95–106.
4. Papachristous D, Fortner J. Comparison of lymphedema following incontinuity and discontinuity groin dissection. *Ann Surg* 1977;185:13–6.
5. Carter BJ. Women's experiences of lymphedema. *Oncol Nurs Forum* 1997;24(5):875–82.
6. Foldi E, Foldi M, Clodius L. The lymphedema chaos: a lancet. *Ann Plast Surg* 1989;22:505–15.
7. Stillwell GK, Redford J, Krusen F. Further studies on the treatment of lymphedema. *Arch Phys Med Rehabil* 1957;38:435–41.
8. Tinkham RG, Stillwell GK. The role of pneumatic pumping devices in the treatment of postmastectomy lymphedema. *Arch Phys Med Rehabil* 1965;193–7.
9. International Society of Lymphology. Consensus document: the diagnosis and treatment of lymphedema. *Lymphology* 1995;28(3):113–7.
10. Education programs leading to qualifications as a physical therapist. *Phys Ther* 1996;76:1352–61.
11. Schulman RS. Statistics in plain english with computer applications. New York: Van Nostrand Reinhold, 1992:110–1.

APPENDIX A.
Lymphedema Questionnaire

Directions: Please circle yes or no for each question. Additional comments may be written in the margins. Related to what is provided in your program's curriculum:

Questions on General Anatomy and Physiology of the Lymphatic System

1. Do you teach the anatomy of the lymphatic system?	Y	N
2. Do you teach the physiology of the lymphatic system?	Y	N
3. Do you teach the pathophysiology of the lymphatic system?	Y	N

Questions on Specific Anatomy and Physiology of the Lymphatic System

4. Do you teach the anatomical components of an initial lymphatic capillary?	Y	N
5. Do you teach the anatomical components of a lymphangion?	Y	N
6. Do you teach your students the characteristics of a lymphotome?	Y	N
7. Do you teach your students the innervation of the lymphatic system?	Y	N
8. Do you discuss the role of the lymphatic system in maintaining the body's homeostasis using Starling's hypothesis?	Y	N

Questions on Pathogenesis of Lymphedema

9. Do you teach the difference between edema and lymphedema?	Y	N
10. Do you discuss the different causes of lymphedema?	Y	N
11. Do you describe to your students the different types of lymphedema?	Y	N
12. Do you list and describe the different grades of lymphedema?	Y	N
13. Do you review the guidelines to prevent lymphedema after surgery?	Y	N

Questions on Traditional Treatment Techniques for Lymphedema

14. Do you teach your students to use a compression pump to manage lymphedema?	Y	N
15. Do you teach your students to use compression pump pressures less than or equal to 45 mmHg?	Y	N
16. Do you teach your students to use compression pump pressures greater than 80 mmHg?	Y	N
17. Do you review the precautions and contraindications when using a compression pump for lymphedema?	Y	N
18. Do you teach your students to instruct the patient to elevate the extremity during the acute phase of lymphedema to reduce limb volume?	Y	N
19. Do you teach your students to instruct the patient to elevate the extremity during the chronic phase of lymphedema to reduce limb volume?	Y	N
20. Do you teach your students how to measure a patient for a compression garment?	Y	N
21. Do you teach your students to order a compression garment upon initial evaluation of the patient?	Y	N
22. Do you teach your students to order a compression garment at the end of physical therapy intervention for lymphedema (i.e., discharge)?	Y	N

Questions on Innovative Treatment Techniques for Lymphedema

23. Do you describe the different components of complex physical therapy (CPT) or complex lymphatic therapy (CLT)?	Y	N
24. Do you teach your students skin care techniques to minimize infections of the edematous limb?	Y	N
25. Do you teach your students compression bandaging using low-stretch bandages to manage lymphedema?	Y	N
26. Do you teach your students compression bandaging using high-stretch bandages (i.e., Ace bandages®) to manage lymphedema?	Y	N
27. Do you teach your students to exercise the patient with some form of external compression (i.e., compression bandages/compression garment)?	Y	N
28. Do you teach your students to exercise the patient without any form of external compression?	Y	N
29. Do you review the physiological effect caused by compression bandaging/compression garment?	Y	N
30. Do you teach/demonstrate to your students manual lymph drainage (massage)?	Y	N
31. Do you review the physiological mechanism that causes limb reduction using manual lymph drainage?	Y	N
32. Do you teach your students how to calculate limb volume to monitor the patient's progress?	Y	N
33. Are your students given any information regarding the research of:		
Foldi (Germany)	Y	N
Leduc (Belgium)	Y	N
Casley-Smith (Australia)	Y	N
Boris (USA)	Y	N

Lymphedema: Patient and Provider Education

Current Status and Future Trends

Carolyn D. Runowicz, M.D.

Division of Gynecologic Oncology, Department of Obstetrics, Gynecology, and Women's Health, Albert Einstein College of Medicine and Montefiore Medical Center, Bronx, New York.

BACKGROUND. The majority of patients schedules for breast surgery or radiation therapy for breast carcinoma do not receive basic information about the risk of lymphedema or its treatment.

METHODS. A review of the literature documenting patient and provider education on the risk, prevention and treatment of lymphedema was undertaken.

RESULTS. Formal education about lymphedema is not a part of the training of most medical and allied health professionals. Thus, patients do not receive information about the risk, prevention, or treatment of lymphedema.

CONCLUSIONS. Educational strategies for patients and providers need to be developed and implemented. *Cancer* 1998;83:2874–6.
© *1998 American Cancer Society.*

KEYWORDS. lymphedema, educational strategies, patient and provider education.

The incidence of upper extremity lymphedema varies from 2% to 40% for women with breast carcinoma who have been treated with surgery, radiation therapy, or both.[1] The reasons for the wide range of incidence rates are related to 1) limited physician knowledge about lymphedema, 2) lack of a universal standard of measurement, 3) lack of a standard definition, 4) prolonged course of development, 5) lack of continued patient contact with the surgeon or radiation oncologists or both, and 6) trivialization of lymphedema as a serious adverse outcome.

Studies document that the majority of patients do not receive basic information about the risk of lymphedema when they are counselled at their initial encounter about their therapeutic options.[2] Furthermore, once lymphedema is diagnosed, patients receive conflicting information. Because there is no cure, patients may feel an abandonment by the medical profession.[3] The presence of lymphedema is a constant reminder of their disease, with economic, physical, and psychosocial sequelae.

Patient education can be divided into three phases: 1) Prior to surgery or radiation, a verbal and written informed consent about the risk of lymphedema, preventive measures, and the potential physical emotional, and economic consequences of lymphedema needs to be given to the patient by the health care provider. 2) Postoperatively, the patient should be educated and counselled about the acute swelling and pain associated with surgery. The patient needs to be given a written set of instructions that include range-of-motion exercises to facilitate recovery. Breast carcinoma patients who comply with instructions on skin care and exercise following surgery show significantly lower incidences of lymphedema.[4] It should be stressed that life-long adherence to the regimen is indicated, because lymphedema

Presented at the American Cancer Society Lymphema Workshop, New York, New York, February 20–22, 1998.

Address for reprints: Carolyn D. Runowicz, M.D., Director, Division of Gynecologic Oncology, Albert Einstein College of Medicine and Montefiore Medical Center, 1695 Eastchester Road, Suite 601, Bronx, New York 10461.

Received July 2, 1998; accepted August 20, 1998.

TABLE 1
Early Recognition of Lymphedema: Signs and Symptoms

Numbness
Tightness
Stiffness
Pain, aching, or heaviness
Redness
Decreased strength
Infection

TABLE 2
Preventing Lymphedema[a]

Avoid injury and infection
  Avoid venipuncture or intravenous infusions
  Wear gardening and cooking gloves and thimbles for sewing
  Suntan gradually, if at all
  Use sunscreen
  Avoid extreme temperatures, e.g., ice packs, heating pads
Avoid constrictive pressure
  Do not use blood pressure cuff or tourniquet
  Wear loose jewelry
Watch for signs of infection, e.g., redness, pain, heat, swelling, fever
Other activities
  Heavy exercise
  Lifting heavy weights or objects
  Avoid letting the arm dangle for long periods of time, e.g., airplane travel

[a] Modified from NIC/PDQ physician statement: Lymphedema—Patient Teaching Guide.

TABLE 3
Patient and Provider Resources

American Cancer Society
National Lymphedema Network
Lymphedema International Network
Oncology Nursing Society
International Society of Lymphology
National Breast Cancer Coalition
National Alliance of Breast Cancer Organizations
American Congress of Rehabilitation Medicine

can develop as late as 15 years or more after surgery. The patient also needs to be educated about the early signs and symptoms of lymphedema to promote its early recognition (Table 1). 3) Finally, for the patient with lymphedema, educational strategies need to be developed to set realistic treatment and outcome goals. The educational process should be aimed at reducing frustration for both the patient and the provider. It should be clear that the goal for lymphedema therapy is to preserve or restore function and cosmesis and will not be curative. Providers need to be educated about the available treatment modalities and support groups so that they can refer patients appropriately. Patients need to be given lists of support and treatment groups to facilitate the appropriate management of lymphedema.

Although there is a long list of proscribed activities, these lists are not evidence based (Table 2). However, until research determines that these activities are safe, it is advisable to provide these lists to patients with the understanding that some of these activities may result in a marked life-style change for some patients. Thus, it is extremely important that patients understand that this list of activities is based more on intuition than on science. Given this information, patients can decide with their health care providers what will work for their individual life styles. Table 3 lists resource organizations that can provider support for both patients and providers.

For health care providers, the educational process should begin in medical school and continue throughout medical training, particularly in those disciplines with patients at risk for the development of lymphedema. Education about the etiopathogenesis of lymphedema and its prevention, assessment, and treatment needs to be formalized and included in existing curricula and textbooks of allied health care professionals as well. Physical therapists need to become skilled providers.

In the United Kingdom, a project was funded by the Department of Health to develop, implement, and evaluate guidelines for the management of breast carcinoma-related lymphedema.[5] This involved the organization of a consensus conference with a multidisciplinary panel of experts, an extensive literature review, the creation of clinical guidelines, and a pilot study to implement and evaluate these guidelines. These guidelines included an educational component aimed at the patient and providers with respect to prevention, assessment, and treatment. There was high compliance to the guidelines. Preventive advice was taken seriously by the patients. A pilot outcome evaluation for patients with lymphedema revealed that the majority of patients experienced an improved outcome, although the number of patients was small. The authors comment that this project highlights the importance of raising awareness of lymphedema through the development and utilization of research-based, patient-centered guidelines.[5]

The education of patients and providers is essential to raise awareness of lymphedema and to promote research into the etiopathogenesis and therapy of this potentially debilitating condition. Lymphedema is not a priority in the curricula of medical professionals. Until there is widespread recognition about lymphedema among patients and health care professionals, there will continue to be a trivialization of this disease process and conflicting treatment information. Lack of education is a serious barrier to the prevention, diagnosis, and treatment of lymphedema.

REFERENCES

1. Logan V. Incidence and prevalence of lymphoedema: A literature review. *J Clin Nurs* 1995;4:213–19.
2. Woods M. Patient's perceptions of breast cancer related lymphoedema. *Eur J Cancer Care* 1993;2:125–8.
3. Carter BJ. Women's experience of lymphedema. *Oncol Nurs Forum* 1997;24:875–82.
4. Getz DH. The primary, secondary and tertiary nursing intervention of lymphedema. *Cancer Nurs* 1985;8:177–84.
5. Kirshbaum M. The development, implementation and evaluation of guidelines for the management of breast cancer related lymphoedema. *Eur J Cancer Care* 1996;5:246–51.

Workgroup I

Treatment of the Axilla with Surgery and Radiation—Preoperative and Postoperative Risk Assessment

A. Marilyn Leitch, M.D. (Co-Chair)
Allen G. Meek, M.D. (Co-Chair)
Robert A. Smith, Ph.D. (Rapporteur)
Marvin Boris, M.D.*
Pierre Bourgeois, M.D., Ph.D.
Susan Higgins, M.D.*
Peter I. Pressman, M.D.*
John Stevens, M.D.*
Randy E. Stevens, M.D.*

* Workgroup participant.

Presented at the American Cancer Society Lymphedema Workshop, New York, New York, February 20–22, 1998.

Address for reprints: Robert A. Smith, Ph.D., American Cancer Society, Inc., 1599 Clifton Rd. NE, Atlanta, GA 30329.

Received October 26, 1998; accepted October 28, 1998.

I. Axillary lymph node dissection (ALND) is currently the standard of care in the management of invasive breast carcinoma.

Lymphedema of the arm is caused by treatment of the axilla with surgery or radiation, and the risk is increased when both modalities are applied to the axilla.[1] Is axillary dissection always necessary in the treatment of breast carcinoma? It was the opinion of the members of Workshop I that some lesions may not require ALND. Furthermore, lymphatic mapping and sentinel lymph node biopsy is a new technique that may obviate the need for ALND and thus avoid its morbidity in certain clinically lymph node negative patients. Clinically lymph node positive and sentinel lymph node positive patients will require ALND for staging and local treatment.

Recommendations

ALND can be avoided in certain cases in which the lesions are low risk, such as ductal carcinoma in situ (DCIS) and certain T1 lesions.[2,3] For those patients for whom ALND is indicated, new surgical approaches, as well as greater care and attention to detail with current approaches, may reduce the risk of posttreatment lymphedema. A promising new approach, and an alternative to ALND, is lymphatic mapping and sentinel lymph node biopsy. In this procedure, the sentinel lymph node is defined as the first lymph node most likely to drain the primary tumor, and thus the first site of metastasis. This lymph node is identified with a mapping procedure that identifies the path of lymphatic drainage after a peritumoral injection of isosulfan blue dye and/or a radiolabeled sulfur colloid. If the "sentinel" lymph node is negative for metastasis, proponents argue that the likelihood of lymph node involvement is low and additional ALND is not necessary. Early results confirm the low likelihood (0–5%) of additional lymph node involvement if the sentinel lymph nodes are negative.[4–6] At this time, sentinel lymph node biopsy technique cannot be casually offered to all breast carcinoma patients. Surgeons who perform this operation should be specifically trained and have a team of physicians in nuclear medicine and pathology available to maximize the efficacy of the procedure. Currently, trained teams of physicians to perform the procedure are not available in all communities throughout the country. Also, the data reported so far on the technique is based on patients undergoing sentinel lymph node biopsy followed by axillary dissection. There is no published data on outcomes for patients undergoing sentinel lymph node biopsy without completion of axillary dissection. The incidence of lymphedema after sentinel lymph node biopsy is unknown, especially in the context of breast conservation in which radiation may overlap the biopsied axilla. Sentinel lymph node biopsy that removes multiple lymph nodes will potentially be associated with a greater risk of lymphedema than when 1 or 2 lymph nodes are removed.

Patients should be informed of the lack of long term follow-up data regarding the incidence of lymphedema and local failure for patients who undergo sentinel lymph node biopsy. Prior to undergoing sentinel lymph node biopsy, patients should be advised of the investigational issues still to be addressed, and they should be registered in clinical trials after giving informed consent.

For those patients who are managed with standard ALND, greater attention must be given to the technical aspects of surgery and radiation to reduce the risk of lymphedema. A greater extent of surgery is associated with increased risk of lymphedema. Because Level I–II ALND is accepted for accurate staging, Level III dissections can be avoided in most patients.[7,8] The surgeon should dissect inferior to the axillary vein and avoid removal of the pectoralis minor muscle. Avoidance of postoperative infection, which can contribute to edema, is extremely important. The axilla should be drained to avoid seroma formation that requires repeated aspiration, which can increase the risk of infection. The drain should be removed promptly when the output is significantly reduced, because the longer dwell time of drains can also increase the risk of infection.

Radiation planning should take into account the extent of axillary surgery. It is desirable to mark the area of dissection with clips to assist the radiation oncologist in planning the field of radiation. The axilla that is dissected should not be radiated unless the risk of regional recurrence is high, such as with macroscopic residual disease or N2 disease. Conventional breast radiation fields encompass portions of the low axilla in many patients. Therefore, radiation fields should be designed in a more conformal manner to avoid this treatment of the axilla. In breast conservation therapy without intention to treat the axilla, computerized 3D planning with CT is critical.

If radiotherapy to the axilla is indicated, it is recommended to use conventional fractions (1.8–2 gray) of megavoltage radiation. Total doses no greater than 45–50 gray are preferred. Sparing the skin at the top of the shoulder allows for collateral lymphatic drainage. If supraclavicular radiation is given, it is desirable to spare as much skin as possible. Postmastectomy radiation should be individualized according to risk of relapse based on initial pathologic findings. Locally advanced breast carcinoma, which frequently requires extensive surgery and radiation, should be approached with prospective multidisciplinary treatment planning, because lymphedema is a common sequela of treatment.

II. There is interest in noninvasive techniques to evaluate the status of the axillary lymph nodes and to assess lymphatic drainage of the arm and breast.

Positron emission tomography scanning may reveal metastatic disease in the axilla but as yet is not sufficiently sensitive to define micrometastases. Radiolabeled monoclonal antibody can also identify involved lymph nodes, but its reliability is not known.

Lymphoscintigraphy can demonstrate the lymphatic pathways from the arm and breast. This will allow evaluation of the extent of disruption of lymphatics by surgery and radiation of the axilla and assessment of the results of complete decongestive therapy with respect to new collaterals for drainage.

Recommendations

Because noninvasive techniques are not yet reliable for staging the axilla, further research should be done to improve resolution. Lymphoscintigraphy could be performed pre- and posttreatment prospectively in a study to assess the impact of ALND and radiation on lymphatics. These studies could help elucidate issues related to the mechanisms of complex lymphedema problems and the efficacy of various therapeutic interventions.

III. In their routine follow-up, clinicians may fail to evaluate for early lymphedema when treatment is more successful.

Recommendations

Clinicians should focus on patient symptoms and signs and respond promptly to patient complaints to insure early referral to a professional who treats lymphedema. Pre- and postoperative measurements may be useful in the assessment of early lymphedema.

IV. There are many issues regarding lymphedema related to breast carcinoma treatment that are unresolved and require directed research.

Recommendations

All clinical trials of breast carcinoma treatment should include lymphedema as an additional endpoint. An important element of this goal is the development of a standardized method of measuring edema. It is important to determine whether it will be useful in treatment planning to document the pathways of lymphatic drainage of the breast and axilla, i.e., with imaging lymphoscintigraphy using two different isotopes preoperatively. Even though sentinel lymph node technique is very promising, conventional patient outcomes must be documented, especially with respect to lymphedema.

REFERENCES

1. Larson D, Weinstein M, Goldberg I, et al. Edema of the arm as a function of the extent of axillary surgery in patients with stage I–II carcinoma of the breast treated with primary radiotherapy. *Int J Radiat Oncol Biol Phys* 1986;12:1575–82.
2. Wood WC. Should axillary dissection be performed in patients with DCIS? *Ann Surg Oncol* 1995;2:193–4.
3. Silverstein MJ, Gierson ED, Waisman JR, et al. Axillary lymph dissection for T1a breast carcinoma: is it indicated? *Cancer* 1994;73:664–7.
4. Giuliano A, Jones RC, Brennan M, Statman R. Sentinel lymphadenectomy in breast cancer. *J Clin Oncol* 1997;15: 2345–50.
5. Albertini JJ, Lyman GH, Cox C, Yeatman T, Reintgen DS, et al. Lymphatic mapping and sentinel node biopsy in the patient with breast cancer. *JAMA* 1996;276:1818–22.
6. Veronesi U, Pogonelli G, Galimberti V, et al. Sentinel node biopsy to avoid axillary dissection in breast cancer with clinically negative nodes. *Lancet* 1997;349:1864–7.
7. Winchester DP, Cox JD. Standards for breast conservation treatment. *CA Cancer J Clin* 1992;42:134–62.
8. Foster RS. The biologic and clinical significance of lymphatic metastases in breast cancer. *Surg Oncol Clin North Am* 1996;5:79–104.

Workgroup II

Patient Education—Pre- and Posttreatment

Carolyn D. Runowicz, M.D. (Co-Chair)
Steven D. Passik, Ph.D. (Co-Chair)
Danette Hann, Ph.D.* (Rapporteur)
Anthony Berson, M.D.*
Helena Chang, M.D., Ph.D.*
Kay Makar, R.D., M.P.H.*
Roberta Moss, M.P.H.*
Janet Osuch, M.D.*
Jeanne D. Petrek, M.D.*
Anne-Marie Vaillant-Newman, P.T.*

*Workgroup participant.

Presented at the American Cancer Society Lymphedema Workshop, New York, New York, February 20–22, 1998.

Address for reprints: Robert A. Smith, Ph.D., American Cancer Society, Inc., 1599 Clifton Rd. NE, Atlanta, GA 30329.

Received October 26, 1998; accepted October 28, 1998.

The workgroup affirmed the importance of pre- and posttreatment education about lymphedema for women who are treated for breast cancer. There is anecdotal evidence that many breast cancer patients who have developed lymphedema were unaware of the risk, symptoms, and potentially protective measures. Pre- and posttreatment education is important because early signs of lymphedema may not be noticed, or the significance may not be appreciated, leading to delays in initiation of treatment and potentially avoidable progression. Further, as treatment advances offer the potential to reduce the risk of lymphedema, breast cancer patients should have the opportunity to make informed decisions about treatment regimens when options exist. The workgroup reached the following conclusions and recommendations:

I. PRETREATMENT PATIENT EDUCATION

A. Pretreatment education should be accurate and evidence based;

B. Pretreatment education interventions should be aimed at awareness about the risks of lymphedema and set the stage for posttreatment education. Posttreatment education should focus on prevention and symptom awareness. There should be information, verbal and written, available to patients and the caregiver spouse/family member about the risks, consequences, prevention, and management of lymphedema;

C. There is a need for reliable and accessible information resources, such as the American Cancer Society, National Cancer Institute, and others, to provide educational information in various forms (electronic, print, etc.) about lymphedema to patients;

D. Education interventions should be appropriate to the medical setting and culturally sensitive to the target population;

E. Patients should be encouraged to obtain treatment from surgeons and radiation therapists most experienced in breast cancer treatment and thereby aware of treatment-related lymphedema.

II. Posttreatment Patient Education

A. Post-treatment education should include information about factors associated with the development of lymphedema. Educational intervention should include a definition and explanation of lymphedema, and the reasons for various hand and arm precautions which should be described in terms of evidence-based importance. The education intervention should be formulated in a positive manner so that the patient's sense of control is enhanced.

B. Patients should be given practical advice on how to avoid situations associated with increased risk of lymphedema, and what to do if these circumstances are encountered (i.e., what to do if the skin is broken on the affected arm). Instruction should also be given on how to recognize early signs of lymphedema;

C. Patients should be reassured that lymphedema is not associated with breast cancer recurrence.

D. Patients and providers should be encouraged to adopt a practical, common sense approach towards recommendations for avoiding lymphedema, especially since forbidden and encouraged activities are not always evidence-based. Providers also should acknowledge the fact that some messages are conflicting, i.e., "Do not exercise, but lose weight." Patients should be informed that these recommendations for risk reduction often are based on anecdotes, but are physiologically consistent, and, where conflicts exists patients should try and find a common ground until better evidence is available.

E. Educational interventions should include spouse/family or caregiver;

F. Educational interventions should address psychosocial aspects of lymphedema (i.e., self-blame, emotional distress) and also should be culturally sensitive.

III. Education Interventions for Patients who Develop Lymphedema

A. Patients should be encouraged to have a comprehensive evaluation by professionals who are experienced in treating lymphedema;

B. Patients should have access to educational materials that provide information on available treatment modalities and the evidence for their efficacy, as well as lists of resources (treatment centers, support groups);

C. Patients should be educated as to realistic goals for management of lymphedema and given specialized training in lymphedema prevention;

D. Patients should be educated about acute management of lymphedema, as well as need for self-maintenance of the stable, but chronic form of lymphedema.

IV. Recommendations for Research and Funding

A. There is a need to develop pretreatment counseling and educational strategies, and to evaluate their efficacy based on (a) retention of information over subsequent periods of time; and (b) patient satisfaction, i.e., confidence about decisions and practices related to quality of life, etc. The evaluation of risk associated with discouraged posttreatment exposures (i.e., vein puncture in the at-risk arm) could be effectively studied in women who have had bilateral mastectomy and thus have no practical alternative.

B. Posttreatment educational strategies need to be developed and evaluated in terms of efficacy of (a) avoidance of risk-related behavior; (b) early recognition of symptoms; (c) prompt care-seeking behavior; and (d) the impact of posttreatment patient education on patients' physical and psychosocial outcomes.

C. There is a critical need for a better understanding of the natural course of this disease, and therefore registries should be developed to follow patients in order to gather information about the risk, onset, and characteristics of post-treatment lymphedema.

D. Breast cancer patients and their providers need guidelines to assess the quality of available interventions and treatment centers.

E. There is a need for a comprehensive literature review of European studies of the various treatment modalities.

F. An available and cost-effective opportunity for prospective research on lymphedema exists in current breast cancer treatment studies. The workgroup recommended that a lymphedema surveillance component should be added to prospective clinical trials now beginning—e.g., chemotherapy trials, as a method of encouraging relatively inexpensive, but potentially lengthy lymphedema studies.

Workgroup III

Diagnosis and Management of Lymphedema

Stanley G. Rockson, M.D. (Co-Chair)
Linda T. Miller, P.T. (Co-Chair)
Ruby Senie, Ph.D. (Rapporteur)
Michael J. Brennan, M.D.*
Judith R. Casley-Smith, M.D., Ph.D.*
Ethel Földi, M.D.*
Michael Földi, M.D.*
Gail L. Gamble, M.D.*
Renato G. Kasseroller, M.D.*
Albert Leduc, Ph.D.*
Robert Lerner, M.D.*
Peter S. Mortimer, M.D.*
Sandra A. Norman, Ph.D.*
Chester L. Plotkin, M.D.*
Margaret E. Rinehart-Ayres, Ph.D., P.T.*
Arnold L. Walder, M.D., Ph.D.*

* Workgroup participant.

Presented at the American Cancer Society Lymphedema Workshop, New York, New York, February 20–22, 1998.

Address for reprints: Robert A. Smith, Ph.D., American Cancer Society, Inc., 1599 Clifton Rd. NE, Atlanta, GA 30329.

Received October 26, 1998; accepted October 28, 1998.

The purpose of this workshop was to derive a consensus statement regarding the diagnosis and treatment of lymphedema following breast carcinoma therapy. The need for such a position statement arises, on the one hand, from a tendency toward therapeutic neglect of this rather prevalent disorder[1] and, on the other, from the recognition that there are currently several broadly practiced schools of lymphedema therapy. In practice, the treatment methods that are promulgated are not always consonant with one another. Thus, it is important to emphasize greater physician awareness of this condition and its prompt recognition, as well as to promote universally applicable approaches to disease management. Several important concepts arose from the workshop discussions: the importance of the patient's subjective presentation with early changes in the trunk or upper extremity, which may presage the clinician's ability to document lymphatic dysfunction objectively; the importance of early management of patients during the first months after breast carcinoma therapy; and the importance of a multidisciplinary approach to the therapy of lymphedema, with differentiation among those modalities that achieve volume reduction of the involved limb from those that maintain long term beneficial therapeutic effects.

RECOMMENDATIONS

Diagnosis

In most cases, the diagnosis of lymphedema following breast carcinoma therapy will be established on the basis of clinical criteria. In this regard, it is important to underscore the value of the patient's subjective awareness of the symptoms or physical changes that accompany the appearance of lymphedema. These subjective complaints may herald the presence of pathology and may, at times, precede the ability of the clinician to detect objective changes of lymphedema on the physical examination. Early detection of pathology can promote the prompt institution of educational and other interventions. Special considerations should apply to symptoms reported by patients during the first 12 weeks following cancer therapy vide infra (v.i.).

In addition to subjectively perceived swelling of the involved extremity, patients may report such sensations as "fullness," "tightness," or "heaviness" of the limb, shoulder girdle, or thoracic regions. All such symptomatic concerns are potentially worthy of attention in these patients and should not be ignored; specifically, any new presentation of pain and immobility of the limb or the shoulder girdle should be promptly evaluated.

In addition to noting the patient's spontaneous complaints,

symptoms of early lymphedema should be actively questioned by the clinician at each evaluation of the patient following breast carcinoma therapy. The patient should not perceive the clinician to be indifferent to the psychosocial, cosmetic, or functional impact of this complication of breast carcinoma treatment. Proper attention to the patient's complaints will serve to validate the patients' concerns and will foster future communication of symptoms by the patient to the clinician. Subjective concerns of the patients should be further validated by recording this data in the clinical record, thereby promoting serial assessment of the problem at follow-up visits.

In many cases of early or subtle lymphedema, a presentation with symptoms will prompt the clinician to note and record objective physical findings of lymphedema, thereby establishing the diagnosis. However, in some cases, there might be a discordance between the patient's subjective concerns and the paucity of findings by physical examination. This discordance does not exclude either the diagnosis or the potential for progression of lymphedema. Indeed, the patient's symptoms alone might warrant the institution of early interventions, such as thorough patient education and more frequent clinical follow-up. Such patient presentations also warrant further scientific evaluation, in order to determine the long term prognostic importance of such patterns of early disease with the natural history of the lymphedema that can follow breast carcinoma treatment.

Objectively, the diagnosis of lymphedema will rely most heavily on assessment of the patient by physical examination. In some cases, where the diagnosis remains in question, a laboratory assessment may be warranted, although at this time a thorough physical examination is felt to be the gold standard for the diagnosis of lymphedema. Radioisotope indirect lymphoscintigraphy is considered a valuable supplemental approach to the detection and quantitation of lymphatic dysfunction,[2] but it has its primary application in research. Where doubt exists regarding a clinical diagnosis, lymphoscintigraphy can be helpful as an adjunctive diagnostic tool.

The physical findings of post–breast carcinoma lymphedema can be either subtle or quite pronounced. A partial list of such findings might include any detectable swelling or enlargement of the limb or trunk, with or without pitting; an increase in the thickness of skin folds, either in the axilla or along the length of the involved extremity, including the digits; a change in the texture or consistency of the skin; or an asymmetric increase in the adiposity of the subcutaneous tissues. Special considerations might apply to the physical findings in patients during the first 12 weeks following cancer therapy (v.i.).

A first presentation of upper body edema in the patient following treatment of breast carcinoma might prompt the clinician to consider and exclude other important comorbidities, such as deep vein thrombosis or recurrent, metastatic malignancy with appropriate objective studies. The possible coexistence of lymphedema and venous disease in these patients also warrants strong consideration. Where necessary, objective documentation of a venous component to lymphedema can be sought with such diagnosis tools as venous Doppler ultrasonography[3] and other forms of direct venous imaging.

Future research efforts in the realm of lymphedema diagnosis should be centered around the development of sensitive and specific screening modalities that would be sufficiently reliable and cost-efficient to be made widely available. Further refinement and standardization of lymphoscintigraphic techniques would enhance attempts to measure the degree of lymphatic dysfunction and thereby advance clinical and research efforts in lymphedema.

The First 12 Weeks

Although lymphedema may have its inception during the days and weeks following breast carcinoma therapy, in general, the signs and symptoms during this early posttreatment interval will more likely represent the acute effects of the surgery: most changes will be transient and will resolve with time. However, subjective complaints and objective findings that intensify, rather than diminish, during the healing phase warrant greater concern.

For most such patients, an appropriate intervention during this phase might be limited to objective assessment through physical examination, institution of preventive measures, and education of the patient in the proper care of the extremity to prevent the development or exacerbation of lymphedema. Some patients will require aggressive physical measures during this early phase; most will not. All such patients should be clinically reassessed at an early interval following the completion of healing from cancer therapy.

Future research efforts should be centered around an investigation into the correlation between early posttherapeutic swelling and the ultimate development of lymphedema. In addition, the recommendations for postsurgical activity and the use of the extremity should be reevaluated. While clinical experience dictates that early immobility after surgery might reduce the incidence of postoperative seroma formation, such measures might not be feasible in the current patient-care environment, in which outpatient surgery and prompt hospital discharge are increasingly recommended. In general, early activity following breast carcinoma surgery should optimally be centered around scapulothoracic, elbow, and hand mobility with an active range of motion exercise in the absence of muscular exertion against resistance.

Therapy

During the first 3 months after cancer therapy, a new diagnosis of clear-cut lymphedema may warrant therapeutic intervention. However, in most cases, complex therapy may not be required. It is recommended that all such cases of new, early lymphedema diagnosis engender a routine referral for physical and occupational therapy (PT/TO) evaluation and, if warranted, institution of appropriate physiotherapy.

The treatment of chronic post–breast carcinoma lymphedema is best achieved through the application of multiple modalities. With the recognition that lymphedema therapy is not solely administered by physical therapists, it is recommended that such terms as *complete decongestive physiotherapy* be replaced with the more universally applicable *decongestive lymphatic therapy;* ideally, uniformity of nomenclature will foster communication among the health care professionals who administer therapy for this disease.

Decongestive lymphatic therapy comprises a number of interrelated treatment modalities that are most efficacious when utilized in an interdependent fashion.[4]

- Proper *skin care* will optimize the supple texture of the skin and, with the other components of this therapy, minimize the risk of infection through cutaneous portals of entry;[5]
- *Manual lymphatic therapy* is a specialized form of massage that has been demonstrated to stimulate and direct lymphatic flow, thereby decreasing the edema and fibrous changes of the involved extremity;
- Application of *multilayered low-stretch bandages* (with appropriate padding) is utilized to enhance the effect of muscular activity upon the clearance of lymphatic fluid from the limb;
- *Exercise* can include, but may not be limited to, active range of motion, and should be individuated according to the patient's medical and psychosocial needs and capacity. Exercise is maximally effective when performed while the lymphedematous limb is bandaged. Isometric exercise is of dubious benefit and may, in fact, promote worsening of the edema.

After effective volume reduction has been accomplished through the combined effects of these modalities, ongoing control of edema must be accomplished through the use of *well-fitted compressive garments.* It is generally not helpful to fit these garments prior to the institution of volume-reducing techniques. The compressive garment should be fitted to apply an appropriate range of external pressure, generally between 30 and 60 mmHg. It is recommended that garments be replaced every 3 months to maintain maximal therapeutic benefit.

Other treatment modalities have been advocated for the control of lymphedema and may warrant a role in therapy when used in concert with the aforementioned techniques. These include:

- *Intermittent compression pumps,* which are most efficacious when used adjunctively in manual lymphatic therapy. The use of these sequential gradient pumps in the absence of a multidisciplinary treatment program should be avoided.
- *Drug therapy* of post–breast carcinoma lymphedema is still under evaluation. The routine use of *diuretics* does not appear to be warranted, unless the patient requires such systemic therapy for coattendant morbid conditions.
- *Benzopyrones,* such as coumarin,[6] are not available for routine use in the U.S. at this time. Although *bioflavenoids*[7] are readily available, long term studies have not yet documented the efficacy of this pharmacologic approach. Prophylactic, long term use of systemic *antibiotics* is routinely warranted for these patients. Nevertheless, it is important to recognize that affected individuals are often subject to repeated bouts of cellulitis, lymphangitis, and other soft tissue infections in the involved extremity.[8] Prompt, aggressive use of systemic antibiotic therapy is clearly warranted in such circumstances, and patients and medical personnel must always be vigilant for evidence of new infection. Although the manifestations of infection can be quite fulminant, in some cases the presentation can be surprisingly subtle, provoking little more than some mild increase in the temperature, erythema, tenderness, or volume of the involved extremity.

Ongoing research efforts should be directed toward resolving the unanswered questions regarding the therapy of lymphedema associated with breast carcinoma. Future research should promote resolution of the following issues, among others:

- Determination of the relative efficacy of each of the components of the comprehensive treatment program;
- Determination of the optimal timing for the institution of various existing treatment modalities within the natural history of the disease;
- Assessment of the role of diagnostic evaluation in predicting the applicability of various therapeutic modalities to individual cases or types of lymphedema associated with breast carcinoma;
- Investigation of the role of early detection and aggressive therapy in reducing the severity of lymphedema and its likelihood of progression;
- Investigation of the efficacy of intensive comprehensive therapy in the prevention of infectious complications of lymphedema;
- Assessment of the efficacy of benzopyrones and other pharmacologic agents in the treatment of lymphedema;
- Development and evaluation of maximally efficacious antibiotic stratagems for the treatment of infectious complications of lymphedema.

REFERENCES

1. Schunemann H, Willich N. Secondary lymphedema of the arm following primary therapy of breast carcinoma. *Zentralbl Chir* 1992;117:220–5.
2. Partsch H. Assessment of abnormal lymph drainage for the diagnosis of lymphedema by isotopic lymphangiography and by indirect lymphography. *Clin Dermatol* 1995;13:445–50.
3. Svensson WE, Mortimer PS, Tohno E, Cosgrove DO. Colour Doppler demonstrates venous flow abnormalities in breast cancer patients with chronic arm swelling. *Eur J Cancer* 1994;30A:657–60.
4. Foldi E, Foldi M, Weissleder H. Conservative treatment of lymphedema of the limbs. *Angiology* 1985;36:171–80.
5. Foldi E. Prevention of dermatolymphangioadenities by combined physiotherapy of the swollen arm after treatment of breast cancer. *Lymphology* 1996;29:91–4.
6. Casley-Smith JR, Morgan RG, Piller NB. Treatment of lymphedema of the arms and legs with 5,6-benzo-[]-pyrone. *N Engl J Med* 1993;329:1158–63.
7. Piller NB, Morgan RG, Casley-Smith JR. A double-blind, cross-over trial of O-(beta-hydroxyethyl) rutosides (benzopyrones) in the treatment of lymphedema of the arms and legs. *Br J Plast Surg* 1988;41:444–5.
8. Mallon EC, Ryan TJ. Lymphedema and wound healing. *Clin Dermatol* 1994;12:89–93.

Workgroup IV

Lymphedema Treatment Resources—Professional Education and Availability of Patient Services

Darlene R. Walley, Ph.D. (Co-Chair)
Elizabeth Augustine, M.S., P.T. (Co-Chair)
Debbie Saslow, Ph.D. (Rapporteur)
Sherry Bailey*
Eunice Jeffs, R.N.*
Bonnie Lasinski, M.A., P.T.*
JoAnn Plotkin*
Maye Walker*

* Workgroup participant.

Presented at the American Cancer Society Lymphedema Workshop, New York, New York, February 20–22, 1998.

Address for reprints: Robert A. Smith, Ph.D., American Cancer Society, Inc., 1599 Clifton Rd. NE, Atlanta, GA 30329.

Received October 26, 1998; accepted October 28, 1998.

Although estimates vary on both the incidence and prevalence of lymphedema related to breast carcinoma treatment, even at the lowest estimate it is a serious public health problem. Lymphedema is a barrier to recovery and rehabilitation from breast carcinoma treatment for a significant number of women today, and will be for a significant number of women who will develop this disease. A common theme heard at the Public Forum that preceded the American Cancer Society Lymphedema Workshop was that health care providers are poorly informed about this disease and therefore commonly do not recognize early symptoms. Providers are also poorly informed about the range of treatment options, which treatment may be most appropriate for the patient, and the availability of treatment in their community. Even if a patient's physician is responsive to signs and symptoms, often they face the vexing challenge of identifying appropriate resources in the community. This workgroup concluded that there was a critical need to provide guidance about lymphedema to health care providers, insurers, and breast carcinoma survivors, especially regarding its early signs and symptoms. There is also a critical need to increase the availability of treatment resources.

I. GUIDANCE

A. Currently, little emphasis is placed on awareness, recognition, or treatment of lymphedema among physicians (gatekeepers), allied health professionals, and insurers.

Recommendation

The American Cancer Society and other appropriate organizations should write an impact statement to disseminate to health care professional organizations, requesting that they each develop clinical practice guidelines that focus on education and recognition of lymphedema that occurs after breast carcinoma treatment. The guidelines will need to cover different treatment needs as well as recognition of lymphedema as a disease (rather than a condition or symptom).

B. Lymphedema is not a priority within the curricula of medical professionals.

Recommendation

Lymphedema case studies should be included in grand rounds, continuing medical education courses, and graduate medical education. Research is needed to determine the best format and content for how to educate health professionals. Cancer-related lymphedema should be incorporated into differential edema diagnosis, e.g., cardiac, venous, etc. The different educational needs of physicians and physical therapists must be addressed.

C. There is insufficient access to good educational materials and textbooks published in English.
Recommendation
Suppliers and authors of medical texts published in English should be contacted about the need for professional education about lymphedema. In addition, efforts should focus on the inclusion of these materials in graduate medical education and their availability in bookstores.

D. There are no guidelines or certification to assure that specific treatments or treatment facilities meet state-of-the-art criteria. It is unclear which body should be responsible for certification.
Recommendation
A multidisciplinary task force should be assembled to establish certification guidelines and determine how they should be implemented and enforced in a way that conforms to a current American system, e.g., JCHO. In the short term, the basic questions patients could ask to compare the qualifications of alternative treatments or treatment settings should be made more widely available.

E. Patients and their physicians generally do not know where to obtain treatment or how to assess the quality of available treatment resources. At this time, the number of treatment centers is inadequate, and the availability of treatment is limited by geography.
Recommendation
The American Cancer Society and other appropriate organizations should issue and widely disseminate a complete lymphedema resource guide. The proliferation of treatment centers based on involvement of an accreditation group and consensus diagnosis/management guidelines should be encouraged. Independent breast carcinoma care and women's health care centers should be certified for lymphedema treatment to ensure that patients have access to comprehensive care.

F. There is a need for management strategies, based on severity and cost-effectiveness, for patients who present with signs or symptoms of lymphedema.
Recommendation
All health care providers should be fully informed of the risk of lymphedema, basic preventive measures, and signs and symptoms of lymphedema, including subjective perceptions consistent with this disease.

Patients presenting with mild lymphedema should be referred to health care professionals who have been trained to administer treatment (e.g., physical therapists), whereas the most severe cases of lymphedema should be referred to health care professionals who have received postprofessional specialized training in lymphedema management (e.g., physical therapists, occupational therapists, nurses, and physicians).

II. COST/ECONOMIC ANALYSIS
A. Currently, the workshop is unaware of cost/economic analyses of the burden of lymphedema. The absence of these data may contribute to the low priority that lymphedema is given by insurers.
Recommendation
There is a need for investigations and analyses to quantify the costs of treating lymphedema patients. The workshop believes that these costs will likely be substantial and may prove persuasive to policymakers.

III. OVERALL PATIENT INTERVENTION STRATEGY
A. There is no consistent guideline regarding when to interact with patients, including prior to or subsequent to breast carcinoma treatment. The workshop affirmed the importance of patient education regarding the risk of lymphedema, post–breast carcinoma treatment behaviors associated with risk and risk reduction, and recognition of early signs and symptoms.
Recommendation
All patients should be provided with information about lymphedema prior to and after breast carcinoma surgery, including reconstruction. Psychosocial research related to communication of posttreatment risk and living with posttreatment risk is needed, as are data on the incidence of lymphedema following different treatment regimens.

B. Currently, there are no standard intervention strategies for patients with lymphedema and no common goal for treatment outcome, i.e., reduction of symptoms, quality of life, etc. This absence of objective criteria and shared outcome goals is believed to be a factor in poor compliance with treatment regimens and lack of understanding by patients.
Recommendation
The American Cancer Society and other appropriate organizations need to develop an overall intervention strategy, including the involvement of patient support systems. Research is needed that compares costs, efficacy, compliance, and quality of life associated with different intervention strategies.

American Cancer Society Lymphedema Workshop

Supplement to ***Cancer***

Workgroup V

Collaboration and Advocacy

Myrna Candeira (Co-Chair)
William Schuch (Co-Chair)
Laura Greiner (Rapporteur)
Lisa Buckley
Heather Gold, M.A.*
Amy Langer, M.B.A.*
Beverly McKane*
Michele Melin, M.P.P.*
Marsha Oakley, R.N., B.S.N.
Joann Schellenbach*
Anne Schuch*
Saskia R. J. Thiadens, R.N.*
Ginny Thompson*
Carin Upstill, M.P.H.*

* Workgroup participant.

Presented at the American Cancer Society Lymphedema Workshop, New York, New York, February 20–22, 1998.

Address for reprints: Robert A. Smith, Ph.D., American Cancer Society, Inc., 1599 Clifton Rd. NE, Atlanta, GA 30329.

Received October 26, 1998; accepted October 28, 1998.

Collaboration, the process by which organizations work together to address a common mission, can benefit organizations through reduced duplication and maximized resources. It will likely require the collaborative efforts of people and organizations with different skills and strengths to create innovation solutions to complex problems like lymphedema. This workshop was convened because of the potential for collaborative efforts among the many organizations addressing issues related to breast cancer.

The workshop included representatives of the following organizations: National Lymphedema Network, National Alliance of Breast Cancer Organizations, American Cancer Society— New York City Division, California Division and National Home Office, Arm-in-Arm, YWCA of U.S.A., the Susan G. Komen Foundation, Y-ME National Breast Cancer Organization, and Bosom Buddies.

The strongest and overarching recommendation from this work group is a call for collaboration within the medical and scientific community to conduct the research necessary to achieve consensus on a standard definition and identifying signs and symptoms of lymphedema, and standards for treatment and management of lymphedema. This consensus will provide the basis for effective advocacy and collaboration on activities related to lymphedema.

In addition, the group endorsed recommendations in the following areas:

Collaboration and Competition

There is tension between organizations attempting to work together because of competition for visibility, volunteers and fundraising. Groups are working together more closely than in the past, but problems caused by competition still exist at the national and grassroots levels. These problems mean fewer women have access to information and services. It is part of our responsibility to the public to strive for more effective collaboration, while still recognizing the individual missions of the organizations involved.

Recommendations:

- Groups working together should clearly define the goal(s) of their collaborative effort;
- Collaborating organizations should acknowledge that competition exists, identify and acknowledge contentious issues, and develop strategies for addressing conflict;

- Organizations should continuously compare their position(s) on issues to identify points of disagreement, and support a philosophy to "agree to disagree" on certain issues (i.e., different priorities for research funding, etc.) in order to move forward with efforts related to their common goals and areas of agreement.

Future Collaboration

Ongoing collaboration between patient advocacy organizations is critical for quality and effective efforts to solve the problem of lymphedema.

Recommendations:

- A mechanism for collaboration must be developed among all breast cancer stakeholders;
- Additional organizations (beyond those represented here) who have a stake in the issue need to be invited to come to the table;
- Information from breast cancer groups' efforts related to lymphedema should be shared with other cancer advocacy groups (i.e., prostate cancer, etc.) for application to lymphedema issues in general.

Organizational Support for Addressing Lymphedema

Many organizations need to increase their internal awareness of and support for addressing lymphedema. Intraorganizational awareness and buy-in needs to be addressed.

Recommendations:

- Consensus on standards is needed to advocate for awareness and support (see first recommendation).
- Workshop participants should go back to their own organizations and encourage an effort to expand the focus of breast cancer support efforts to include addressing lymphedema in all areas.

Patient and Provider Education

Collaboration needs to take place to more effectively reach patients and providers with information about lymphedema.

Recommendations:

- There is an urgent need for consensus on standardized information to develop fast track professional and public education campaigns;
- Patient advocacy groups should collaborate with professional societies to advance professional education, i.e., publications and training;
- Patient advocacy groups should work with managed care organizations, policy makers and insurance companies to influence favorable reimbursement policies;

- Information should be distributed to support groups, to cultivate participants as advocates to help educate their providers;
- Breast cancer organizations should be prepared to refer women to existing resources on lymphedema through their information delivery vehicles (800 numbers, websites, breast cancer resource listings, etc.).

Informed Consent and Information

It is critical that women receive accurate information before and after treatment about the risk of lymphedema and preventive measures that should be followed.

Recommendation:

- Patient advocacy groups should advocate for written informed consent prior to breast cancer treatment.

Legislative and Patient Advocacy

Agreement on treatment standards is necessary to develop a legislative advocacy platform. The work group agreed that legislative advocacy is a critical strategy in addressing the needs of those living with lymphedema. Issues such as licensure for certification and adequate and fair grievance procedures are important, but again rely on clear quality standards. Grievance procedures are particularly important as long as lymphedema treatment is not widely covered by insurance. "Advocacy" can also be considered from the perspective of patient advocacy. Efforts in this area include strategies for helping women feel empowered to seek out information and participate fully with their health care providers in medical decision making.

Legislative Recommendations:

- Advocate for additional research dollars allocated to lymphedema research within breast cancer research funding.
- Advocate for coverage of industry established standard treatment modalities.

Insurance Recommendation:

- A work group should be formed to develop a model for insurance coverage of lymphedema treatment services (standards consensus needed).

Research and Data

The Workgroup acknowledged that advocacy initiatives are inherently limited by the absence of scientific data on the incidence and prevalence of lymphedema, costs, psychosocial consequences, and the efficacy of different treatment regimens.

Recommendations:

- There is a need for surveillance systems to better understand the epidemiology of lymphedema, and other investigations related to efficacy of various treatments and duration of treatment. These investigations may be both retrospective and prospective. The cost of not treating lymphedema should also be estimated, since these data on disease burden could be persuasive to policy makers and managed care organizations;

- There is a need for psychosocial research related to lymphedema and risk of lymphedema. Investigations should focus on pre- and posttreatment communication recognizing that this is a time when women are dealing with life and death issues of breast cancer;

- Cooperative groups that are doing prospective research on breast cancer should add a lymphedema surveillance component to the existing protocols.

Lymphedema Resource Guide

LYMPHEDEMA ORGANIZATIONS

International Society of Lymphology
The University of Arizona, College of Medicine, Department of Surgery (GS&T), P.O. Box 245063, 1501 N. Campbell Avenue, Tucson, Arizona 85724-5063; (520) 626-6118; http://www.u.arizona.edu/~witte/ISL.htm

Description: The society was established in 1966 and includes over 375 members from 35 countries. The goals of the organization are to further knowledge and research in the field of lymphology and related topics; establish relationships between researchers and clinicians; facilitate personal contact and exchange of ideas among lymphologists; and organize working groups (e.g., lymphology in filariasis, lymphedema treatment, lymphatic imaging, endolymphatic radiotherapy, AIDS-Kaposi sarcoma) or regional chapters.

Lymphedema Foundation
8307 Marbach Road, San Antonio, Texas 78227; (210) 675-5599; http://lymphedemafoundation.org

Description: The foundation was established to support research for the cause, prevention, and treatment of lymphedema; to make information about lymphedema available to physicians, patients, and the public; to educate health care providers and insurers about the need for appropriate care for lymphedema patients; to advocate for patients; and to establish certification standards for lymphedema therapists and facilities.

Lymphoedema Association of Australia
94 Cambridge Terrace, Malvern, S.A. 5061, Australia; 61+(8) 8271-2198; http://www.lymphoedema.org.au

Description: The association was established in 1982 and includes over 2,000 members, 25 percent of whom live in countries outside of Australia. The major goals of the association are to support lymphedema research and its treatment, and to provide information to physicians, therapists and patients.

Lymphovenous Canada
8 Silver Avenue, Toronto, Ontario, Canada M6R 1X8; (416) 533-2428; http://www.lymphovenous-canada.com

Description: The major goal of the organization is to provide objective information on recent developments in research and treatment in lymphedema. It also provides patient referrals for physicians and support groups.

National Lymphedema Network
2211 Post Street, Suite 404, San Francisco, CA 94115-3259; (415) 921-1306; (800) 541-3259 (Information hotline); http://www.lymphnet.org

Description: A nonprofit agency which offers information and education about lymphedema, a referral service to medical and therapeutic treatment centers, and information on locating or establishing local support groups. It publishes the *NLN Newsletter* (quarterly) which contains articles on lymphedema and related topics, including a resource guide of treatment centers, physicians, therapists and suppliers; a listing of over 100 lymphedema support groups, PenPals/NetPals, and special features.

OTHER ORGANIZATIONS ADDRESSING LYMPHEDEMA

American Association of Cardiovascular and Pulmonary Rehabilitation
7611 Elmwood Avenue, Suite 201, Middleton, WI 53562; (608) 831-6989; http://www.aacvpr.org

Description: The mission of the association is to reduce morbidity, mortality, and disability from cardiovascular and pulmonary diseases through education, prevention, rehabilitation and aggressive disease management. Members receive the *Journal of Cardiopulmonary Rehabilitation* and quarterly newsletter.

American Cancer Society
Reach to Recovery; (800) ACS-2345; http://www.cancer.org

Description: A nonprofit organization that provides information and support to breast cancer survivors. The volunteers from this program are women who have had breast cancer and are specially trained to share their knowledge and experiences in a supportive and non-intrusive manner. Ongoing support groups are available to help deal with the challenges of breast cancer. It also provides referrals to local diagnostic and treatment centers.

American Society of Clinical Oncology
225 Reinekers Lane, Suite 650, Alexandria, VA 22314; (703) 299-0150; http://www.asco.org

Description: A nonprofit organization whose membership includes more than 10,000 cancer professionals worldwide. It offers scientific and educational programs and a broad range of other initiatives intended to foster the exchange of information about cancer. The organization serves the needs of the oncology community through a broad range of programs and services and publishes the *Journal of Clinical Oncology*.

II

National Alliance of Breast Cancer Organizations (NABCO)
9 E. 37th Street, 10th Floor, New York, NY 10016;
(800) 719-9154 or (212) 719-0154; http://www.nabco.org

Description: A non-profit organization that is a resource of information about breast cancer and a network of more than 370 organizations that provide detection, treatment and care.

National Breast Cancer Coalition
1707 L Street, NW, Suite 1060, Washington, DC, 20036;
(202) 296-7477; http://www.natlbcc.org

Description: A grassroots action and advocacy network of over 450 organizations that is dedicated to eliminating breast cancer.

National Cancer Institute (NCI)
Cancer Information Center; (800) 4-CANCER;
http://www.nci.nih.gov

Description: A government agency that provides cancer information to people with cancer and their families, the public, and health care professionals. NCI maintains a listing of current clinical trials.

National Coalition for Cancer Survivorship
1010 Wayne Avenue, 5th Floor, Suite 300, Silver Spring, MD 20910; (888) 937-6227 or (301) 650-8868;
http://www.cansearch.org

Description: A network of individuals and organizations that provide cancer support and information.

The Society for Vascular Medicine and Biology
13 Elm Street, Manchester, MA 01944; (978) 526-8330;
http://www.svmb.org

Description: A professional organization which was founded in 1989 to improve the integration of vascular biological advances into medical practice, and to maintain high standards of clinical vascular medicine. Affiliated with the American Venous Forum (www.venous-info.com) which includes more than 225 board-certified vascular surgeons who have an interest in contributing to the management of venous disease. The forum provides an academic colloquium to physicians interested in the research, education, and clinical investigation in the field of venous diseases.

Society for Vascular Nursing
7794 Grow Drive, Pensacola, FL 32414; (888) 536-4SVN;
http://www.svnnet.org

Description: An international association which was established in 1982. The society is dedicated to promoting quality standards in the comprehensive management of persons with vascular disease. The focus is on providing education, fostering clinical expertise, and supporting nursing research. Members receive a newsletter and the *Journal of Vascular Nursing.*

The Susan G. Komen Breast Cancer Foundation
5005 LBJ Freeway, Suite 370, Dallas, TX 75244; (972) 855-1600;
(800) 462-9273 (National toll-free breast care helpline);
http://komen.org and http://breastcancerinfo.com

Description: The mission of the organization is to eliminate breast cancer through promoting research, education, screening, and treatment. It is the largest private funder of research dedicated solely to breast cancer in the United States.

Y-Me National Breast Cancer Hotline
212 West Van Buren, Chicago, IL 60607, (800) 221-2141;
(800) 986-9505 (Spanish); http://www.y-me.org

Description: An organization which provides a national hotline, public meetings and seminars, workshops for professionals, referral service, resource library, teen program, and advocacy. Also publishes a bimonthly newsletter.

LYMPHEDEMA SUPPORT GROUPS
There are over 50 lymphedema support groups throughout the country. Contact your local American Cancer Society for information regarding groups in your area. The following is a listing of groups that offer information via the Internet.

Bosom Buddies Breast Cancer & Lymphedema Support Group
776 Willow Brook Drive #802, Naples, FL 34108-8541;
(941) 514-3845; http://www.go-icons.com/bosombuddies.htm

Breast Cancer Network of Western New York, Inc.
(716) 631-8665;
http://rpci.med.buffalo.edu/departments/breast/rpframe.html

Greater Boston Lymphedema Network
77 Graymore Road, Waltham, MA 02451; (781) 894-2309;
http://208.201.252.102/lsg

The Mid-Atlantic Lymphedema Center
5010 Dorsey Hall Drive, Ellicott City, MD 21042; (800) 845-7525;
http://www.lymphedemacrc.com

National Lymphedema Network Newsletter (lists over 100 lymphedema support groups)
2211 Post Street, Suite 404, San Francisco, CA 94115-3259;
(415) 921-1306; (800) 541-3259 (Information hotline);
http://www.lymphnet.org

Trinity Lymphedema Centers
P.O. Box 1481, Palm Harbor, FL 34682; (800) 585-8057;
http://www.trinitylc.com/support.html

Online Lymphedema Support Groups

http://tile.net/lists/lymphedema.html
Type in the body of your e-mail: SUBSCRIBE LYMPHEDEMA your first name and your last name and send to: listserv@listserv.acor.org

http://www.lifetimetv.com/chat/unmoderated_chats.html
(live online support group)

ONLINE INFORMATION

The following are the top sites for information related to lymphedema.

CancerBACUP
http://www.cancerbacup.org.uk/info/lymphedema.htm

CancerNet (NCI)
http://cancernet.nci.nih.gov/clinpdq/supportive/Lymphedema_Physician.html; http://cancernet.nci.nih.gov/clinpdq/supportive_span/Linfedema.html (Spanish version)

Mayo Clinic (Health Oasis)
http://www.mayohealth.org/mayo/9701/htm/swollen.htm

OncoLink
http://www.oncolink.com/support/lymphedema

Lymphedema Family Study (University of Pittsburgh)
http://www.pitt.edu/~genetics/lymph/lymph.htm

RECOMMENDED READING
Consumer Publications

Breast Cancer Action Ottawa. Lymphedema—a breast cancer legacy. Booklet can be ordered from: Billings Bridge Plaza, P.O. Box 39041, Ottawa, Ont. K1H 1A1 (613) 736-5921. http://infoweb.magi.com/~bcanet.

Dinclaux AJ. Nutritherapy for lymphedema. Desert Hot Springs, CA: E.S.O.P. Publications. http://www.inetad1.com/lymphdma.htm.

Kneece JC. Your breast cancer treatment handbook: Columbia: SC: EduCare, Inc., 1998.

Love S. Dr. Susan Love's breast book. NY: Perseus Press, 1995.

Stumm D. Recovering from breast surgery. Cedar Rapids, IA: Hunter House, 1995.

Swirsky J, Nannery DS. Coping with lymphedema. Garden City Park, NY: Avery Publishing Group, 1998.

Weiss MC, Weiss E. Living beyond breast cancer. NY: Times Books, 1998.

Weissleder H, Schuchardt C. Lymphedema: diagnosis and therapy (2nd ed). Bonn, Germany: Kagerer KommuniKation, 1997. http://home.earthlink.net/~ralphweis.

Professional Publications

Cluzan RV, Pecking AP, Lokiec FM. Progress in lymphology-XIII: proceedings of the Xiiith International Congress of Lymphology (internatio), Paris, France, 29 September–5 October, 1991. NY: Elsevier Science, 1992.

Foldi M, Foldi E, Newell AC. Lymphoedema: methods of treatment and control: a guide for patients and therapists. Portland, OR. Medicina Biologica, 1993.

Harris JR, Lippman ME, Morrow M, Hellman S. Diseases of the breast. New York: Lippincott, 1996.

Kasseroller R, Thrift KM, Fogg DM. Compendium of Dr. Vodder's manual lymph drainage. Portland, OR: Medicina Biologica, 1998.

Olszewski WL. Lymph stasis: pathophysiology, diagnosis, and treatment. Boca Raton, FL: CRC, 1991.

Wittlinger H, Wittlinger G, Kurz I. Textbook of Dr. Vodder's manual lymph drainage. Portland, OR: Medicina Biologica, 1997.

SUPPLIERS OF COMPRESSION GARMENTS AND PUMPS

Barton-Carey Custom Stockings, 26963 Eckel Rd., Suite 303, Perrysburg, OH 43551; (800) 421-0444.

Beiersdorf, Inc. (Jobst® and Elvarex®), 653 Miami Street, Toledo, OH 43605; (800) 537-1063; http://www.beiersdorf-medical.com

Bio Compression Sequential Circulator (Venosan), 120 West Commercial Avenue, Moonachie, NJ 07074; (800) ABC-PUMP; http://woundcare.org/newsvol2n1/ar11a.htm

CBF, 8044 Ray Mears Boulevard, Suite 100, Knoxville, TN 37919; (800) 225-8129.

CircAid Medical Products, Inc., 9323 Chesapeake Drive, Suite B-1, San Diego, CA 92123; (800) CIRCAID; http://www.circaid.com

Conco Medical Co., 481 Lakeshore Pkwy, Rock Hill, SC 29730; (800) 243-2294; http://medicalmag.com/abco_data/conco_medical.html

Freeman Manufacturing Company, P.O. Box J, Surgis, MI 49091; (616) 651-2371; http://www.freemanmfg.com

Healthtronix Medical Equipment, Inc., 811 East Plano Parkway, Suite 111, Plano, TX 75074; (800) 349-9490; http://healthtronix.com

J & C Associates, Inc., 212 High Street, Geneva, NY 14456; (800) 756-7269; http://www.j-c.net

Juzo (Julius Zorn, Inc.), P.O. Box 1088, Cuyahoga Falls, OH 44223; (800) 222-4999; http://www.juzousa.com

Legacy Compression Systems, 1800 NW Market Street, Seattle, Washington 98107; (206) 782-8554; http://www.lymphclinic.com

Medi Stockings & Sleeves, 76 West Seegers Road, Arlington Heights, IL 60005; (800) 633-6334

Mego Afek, Kibbutz Afek 30042, Israel; (972) 4-8784277; http://www.lympha-press.com

Newport Center Orthopedic, 400 Newport Center Drive, Suite 104, Newport Beach, CA 92660; (949) 644-0065

Progressive Motion, 1030 W. Pedregosa St., Santa Barbara, CA 93101; (805) 898-0760; http://www.progressivemotion.com

Sigvaris (Ganzoni), 1119 Hwy 74 South, Peachtree City, GA 30269; (800) 322-7744.

Western Health Care Industries, Inc., 723 Court Street, Jackson, CA 95642; (800) 464-7306; http://www.whcii.com/compress.htm

The W.I.S.E. Center, 510 Oldbridge Turnpike, South River, NJ 08882; (800) 870-6616

TRAINING PROGRAMS FOR LYMPHEDEMA THERAPY

Academy of Lymphatic Studies, 12651 W. Sunrise Blvd., Suite 101, Sunrise, FL 33323; (800) 232-5542; http://www.lymphedemaservices.com

The Casley-Smith School, 94 Cambridge Terrace, Malvern S.A. 5061, Australia; 011-61-8-8271-2198; www.lymphoedema.org.au

The Foldi School, Roesslehofweg 2-6, 79856 Hinterzarten, Germany; 011-49-761-406921; www.foeldiklinik.de

Lymphedema Management LeDuc Method, Post Office Box 79, Woodbury CT 06798; (203) 266-9133

The Vodder School of North America, P.O. Box 5701, Victoria, B.C., Canada V8R 6S8; (250) 598-9862; http://www.vodderschool.com

The agencies, organizations, and corporations represented in this resource guide are not necessarily endorsed by the American Cancer Society. This guide is provided for assistance in obtaining information. There are no current national standards that have been set for the treatment of lymphedema, certification of professionals in the field, or accreditation of lymphedema training courses.